MW00623771

HEALTHCHEQUES

Carbohydrate, Fat & Calorie Guide

Jane Stephenson, RD, CDE
Diane Bader

Fourth Edition

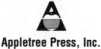

Appletree Press, Inc.
Mankato, Minnesota

Appletree Press, Inc.
151 Good Counsel Drive Suite 125
Mankato, MN 56001

Phone: (507) 345-4848
Fax: (507) 345-3002
Website: www.appletree-press.com

The purpose of *HealthCheques™: Carbohydrate, Fat & Calorie Guide* is to supply authoritative data on the nutritional values of foods in a form for quick and easy reference. The information is not intended as a substitute for treatment prescribed by your physician. Please consult with your licensed health care professional before making any changes to your treatment plan.

CATALOGING-IN-PUBLICATION DATA

Stephenson, Jane, 1960-

HealthCheques™: Carbohydrate, Fat & Calorie Guide / authored by Jane Stephenson and Diane Bader. Mankato, MN : Appletree Press, Inc., © 2012.

132 p. ; 13 cm.

Includes index and bibliographical references.

1. Food—Composition—Tables. 2. Nutrition—Tables. 3. Food—Caloric content—Tables. 4. Food—Cholesterol content—Tables. 5. Food—Fat content—Tables. 6. Food—Carbohydrate content—Tables. 7. Convenience foods—Composition—Tables. I. Title. II. Title: HealthCheques. III. Title: Carbohydrate, fat & calorie guide. IV. Title: Carbohydrate, fat and calorie guide. V. Bader, Diane, 1955-

Summary: Values for calories, carbohydrates, carb choices, protein, fat, saturated fat, cholesterol, sodium, and fiber content are provided for more than 4,500 foods, including 18 fast-food chains. A handy nutrition reference and pocket counter.

ISBN 13:978-1-891011-10-8
ISBN 10:1-891011-10-3

RA 784.S74 2004   613.28   2004103638

Editor: Linda Hachfeld
Graphic Designer, Second, Third & Fourth Editions:
    Kristin Higginbotham, Lorie Giefer
Cover and Book Design: Douglas Allan Graphic Design

Printed in the United States of America

Sincere Thanks

We wish to thank our colleagues and publisher who contributed their time, expertise and inspiration in the development of HealthCheques™: Carbohydrate, Fat & Calorie Guide. We extend a special acknowledgment to Jackie Boucher, MS, RD, CDE, for her endless ideas, encouragement and assistance with the introduction of the book; Bridgett Wagener, RD for co-authoring the first edition of this book; and Nikki Bader and Eva Galvez for their help with the manuscript.

We also thank our families and friends for their patience and understanding during the many hours of research involved in writing this book. Finally, we thank our HealthCheques™ customers who strive to achieve their nutrition and health goals each and every day.

Jane Stephenson, RD, CDE
Diane Bader

Authors

Contents

About This Book

HealthCheques™: Carbohydrate, Fat & Calorie Guide was written as a reference to help you make healthy food choices at home, on the run or in restaurants. It lists the calories, carbohydrate, protein, fat, saturated fat, cholesterol, sodium and fiber content of 4,500 foods and includes carbohydrate choices for persons with diabetes.

The foods in this guide are grouped into easy-to-find categories and then listed alphabetically from A to Z. Within each category you'll find subcategories. For example, under the category of Meats, the subcategories are Beef, Game, Lamb, Pork, Processed & Luncheon Meats and Specialty & Organ Meats. Serving sizes listed for individual foods within a category are consistent for easy comparison. Manufacturer's suggested servings are used in cases when serving sizes varied, such as in the Cereal section. Often two measures are given for foods that are available in more than one portion size; for example, Bagel, blueberry "1 (2 oz.)". Values listed inside parentheses such as Bagel, mini "2 (0.9 oz.)" refer to the value of each item; thus, each of the two mini bagels weigh 0.9 ounces.

Learn how to estimate your daily nutrient goals in three easy steps on page 123. To determine carbohydrate grams and choices by calorie level, please turn to page 124. Use the charts on pages 129 and 130 to estimate the number of calories used during 30 minutes of various activities. In addition, you can track your blood lipid levels (Cholesterol, HDL, LDL and Triglycerides) on pages 125-126.

This comprehensive guide is a terrific tool to help you stay healthy—keep it handy in your purse, pocket, desk drawer or glove compartment.

Abbreviations used in HealthCheques™

BBQ	. . . . .barbecue	**pkg.**	. . . . .package
dk.	. . . . .dark	**pkt.**	. . . . .packet
drmstk.	. . . . .drumstick	**T.**	. . . . .tablespoon
fl. oz.	. . . . . . .fluid ounce	**tsp.**	. . . . .teaspoon
frzn.	. . . . .frozen	**veg.**	. . . . .vegetables
g	. . . . .gram	**w/**	. . . . .with
hmde.	. . . . . .homemade	**w/o**	. . . . . . .without
in.	. . . . .inch	**whip'd**	. . . . .whipped
marg.	. . . . . .margarine	**~**	. . . . .approximately*
mayo.	. . . . . .mayonnaise	**/**	. . . . .or*
mg	. . . . .milligram		
n/a	. . . . .not available		

*Examples:
  Servings per dish = ~2
  jam/jelly = jam "or" jelly

oz.	. . . . .ounce
pc.	. . . . .piece

Nutrient values have been rounded to the nearest calorie, gram or milligram, with the exception of saturated fat values, which are rounded to the nearest 0.5 gram. Apparent inconsistencies may result from rounding off numbers, values may have been obtained from more than one source or samples of the same food, seasonal differences and slight variations among manufacturers.

Nutrient values change as products and recipes are reformulated and reanalyzed. Menu items listed may not be available at all restaurants and nutrient values for fast food restaurants are meant for general informational purposes only. Nutrient values are subject to change; values are current as of 2012. If the information you find on a label differs significantly from the data in this book, please use the label as your guide.

ALCOHOL

ITEM	AMOUNT	CALORIES	CARBOHYDRATE (g)	CARBOHYDRATE CHOICES	PROTEIN (g)	FAT (g)	SATURATED FAT (g)	CHOLESTEROL (mg)	SODIUM (mg)	FIBER (g)
ALCOHOL										
Alabama slammer	4 fl. oz.	325	29	2	0	0	0.0	0	5	0
B-52	4 fl. oz.	403	43	3	1	8	4.5	19	49	0
Bahama mama	6 fl. oz.	253	21	1 ½	0	0	0.0	0	19	0
Beer										
light	12 fl. oz.	99	5	0	1	0	0.0	0	11	0
nonalcoholic	12 fl. oz.	73	14	1	1	0	0.0	0	10	0
regular	12 fl. oz.	143	13	1	1	0	0.0	0	7	0
Black Russian	4 fl. oz.	308	20	1	0	0	0.0	0	4	0
Bloody Mary	8 fl. oz.	127	6	½	2	0	0.0	0	458	0
Bourbon & soda	4 fl. oz.	98	0	0	0	0	0.0	0	18	0
Brandy	1 fl. oz.	64	0	0	0	0	0.0	0	0	0
Brandy Alexander	4 fl. oz.	289	15	1	1	8	5.0	26	16	0
Champagne	4 fl. oz.	80	12	1	0	0	0.0	0	10	0
Cordials/liqueurs, 54 proof	1 fl. oz.	100	13	1	0	0	0.0	0	2	0
Cosmopolitan	6 fl. oz.	225	25	1 ½	0	0	0.0	0	4	0
Daiquiri	6 fl. oz.	316	12	1	0	0	0.0	0	9	0
Fuzzy navel	8 fl. oz.	249	31	2	1	0	0.0	0	2	0
Gimlet	2.5 fl. oz.	146	1	0	0	0	0.0	0	1	0
Gin & tonic	8 fl. oz.	156	8	½	0	0	0.0	0	7	0
Gin fizz	8 fl. oz.	140	6	½	0	0	0.0	0	38	0
Gin/rum/vodka/whiskey										
80 proof	1 fl. oz.	64	0	0	0	0	0.0	0	0	0
86 proof	1 fl. oz.	70	0	0	0	0	0.0	0	0	0
90 proof	1 fl. oz.	73	0	0	0	0	0.0	0	0	0
100 proof	1 fl. oz.	84	0	0	0	0	0.0	0	0	0
Grasshopper	4 fl. oz.	344	31	2	1	7	4.5	24	17	0
Harvey wallbanger	6 fl. oz.	191	18	1	1	0	0.0	0	2	0
High ball	4 fl. oz.	74	0	0	0	0	0.0	0	18	0
Hot buttered rum	4 fl. oz.	142	2	0	0	5	3.5	14	3	0
Hot toddie	8 fl. oz.	113	5	0	0	0	0.0	0	3	0
Hurricane	8 fl. oz.	221	29	2	1	0	0.0	0	5	0
Irish coffee										
w/ whipped cream	8 fl. oz.	126	2	0	1	3	2.0	10	22	0
w/o whipped cream	8 fl. oz.	97	1	0	0	0	0.0	0	4	0
Irish cream	1 fl. oz.	106	6	½	1	5	2.5	11	26	0
Kahlua	1 fl. oz.	100	13	1	0	0	0.0	0	2	0
Kamikaze	4 fl. oz.	225	20	1	0	0	0.0	0	3	0
Long Island iced tea	6 fl. oz.	241	21	1 ½	0	0	0.0	0	36	0
Mai tai	4 fl. oz.	274	26	2	0	0	0.0	0	10	0
Manhattan	2.5 fl. oz.	149	2	0	0	0	0.0	0	2	0

ALCOHOL

ITEM	AMOUNT	CALORIES	CARBOHYDRATE (g)	CARBOHYDRATE CHOICES	PROTEIN (g)	FAT (g)	SATURATED FAT (g)	CHOLESTEROL (mg)	SODIUM (mg)	FIBER (g)
Margarita										
w/ salt	6 fl. oz.	375	24	1 ½	0	0	0.0	0	479	0
w/o salt	6 fl. oz.	375	24	1 ½	0	0	0.0	0	9	0
Martini										
appletini	2.5 fl. oz.	175	8	½	0	0	0.0	0	0	0
chocolate	2.5 fl. oz.	190	8	½	0	0	0.0	0	0	0
pomegranate	2.5 fl. oz.	146	7	½	0	0	0.0	0	2	0
traditional	2.5 fl. oz.	159	0	0	0	0	0.0	0	1	0
Melon ball	8 fl. oz.	212	26	2	1	0	0.0	0	3	0
Mimosa	8 fl. oz.	123	24	1 ½	1	0	0.0	0	9	0
Mint julep	4 fl. oz.	272	7	½	0	0	0.0	0	1	0
Mojito	4 fl. oz.	206	16	1	0	0	0.0	0	24	1
Mudslide	4 fl. oz.	358	26	2	1	8	4.5	19	47	0
Old fashioned	4 fl. oz.	265	8	½	0	0	0.0	0	1	0
Pina colada	6 fl. oz.	328	43	3	1	4	3.0	0	11	1
Rob Roy	2.5 fl. oz.	155	1	0	0	0	0.0	0	2	0
Rum & cola	8 fl. oz.	176	20	1	0	0	0.0	0	5	0
Rusty nail	4 fl. oz.	309	17	1	0	0	0.0	0	3	0
Screwdriver	8 fl. oz.	194	20	1	1	0	0.0	0	2	0
Sex on the beach	6 fl. oz.	215	17	1	0	0	0.0	0	2	0
Singapore sling	6 fl. oz.	173	9	½	0	0	0.0	0	25	0
Slo-screw	8 fl. oz.	194	20	1	1	0	0.0	0	2	0
Sloe gin fizz	8 fl. oz.	124	3	0	0	0	0.0	0	39	0
Tequila Maria	8 fl. oz.	127	6	½	2	0	0.0	0	458	0
Tequila sunrise	6 fl. oz.	219	30	2	1	0	0.0	0	8	0
Toasted almond	4 fl. oz.	278	19	1	2	15	9.5	51	33	0
Tom Collins	8 fl. oz.	148	17	1	0	0	0.0	0	104	0
Whiskey sour	4 fl. oz.	174	15	1	0	0	0.0	0	69	0
White Russian	4 fl. oz.	292	19	1	0	1	1.0	4	8	0
Wine, cooking										
Marsala	2 T.	45	4	0	0	0	0.0	0	190	0
red/white	2 T.	20	3	0	0	0	0.0	0	180	0
sherry	2 T.	29	5	0	0	0	0.0	0	180	0
Wine, table										
dessert, dry	4 fl. oz.	149	5	0	0	0	0.0	0	11	0
dessert, sweet	4 fl. oz.	181	14	1	0	0	0.0	0	11	0
red/rosé	4 fl. oz.	100	3	0	0	0	0.0	0	5	0
sangria	8 fl. oz.	157	21	1 ½	0	0	0.0	0	16	0
sherry, dry	4 fl. oz.	82	2	0	0	0	0.0	0	9	0
white, dry/medium	4 fl. oz.	98	3	0	0	0	0.0	0	6	0
Wine cooler	12 fl. oz.	170	20	1	0	0	0.0	0	29	0
Wine spritzer	8 fl. oz.	95	2	0	0	0	0.0	0	30	0

BEVERAGES

ITEM	AMOUNT	CALORIES	CARBOHYDRATE (g)	CARBOHYDRATE CHOICES	PROTEIN (g)	FAT (g)	SATURATED FAT (g)	CHOLESTEROL (mg)	SODIUM (mg)	FIBER (g)
BEVERAGES										
Café latte										
w/ skim milk	8 fl. oz.	80	12	1	8	1	0.5	5	110	0
w/ whole milk	8 fl. oz.	135	11	1	8	7	4.5	30	105	0
Café mocha, w/ whipped cream										
w/ skim milk	8 fl. oz.	145	20	1	7	6	3.0	38	80	1
w/ whole milk	8 fl. oz.	185	20	1	7	11	6.0	55	80	1
Cappuccino										
w/ skim milk	8 fl. oz.	55	8	½	5	0	0.0	3	70	0
w/ water, flavored mix	8 fl. oz.	60	15	1	0	0	0.0	0	0	0
w/ whole milk	8 fl. oz.	130	10	½	7	7	4.0	28	98	0
Capri Sun®										
25% less sugar	6 fl. oz.	60	16	1	0	0	0.0	0	15	0
regular	6 fl. oz.	90	21	1 ½	0	0	0.0	0	25	0
Roarin' Waters	6 fl. oz.	30	8	½	0	0	0.0	0	15	0
Club soda/seltzer	8 fl. oz.	0	0	0	0	0	0.0	0	57	0
Coconut water	8 fl. oz.	47	12	1	0	0	0.0	0	25	0
Coffee										
brewed/instant	6 fl. oz.	2	0	0	0	0	0.0	0	3	0
flavored mixes	6 fl. oz.	60	10	½	0	2	0.5	0	40	0
Crystal Light®	8 fl. oz.	5	0	0	0	0	0.0	0	35	0
Espresso	3 fl. oz.	2	0	0	0	0	0.0	0	12	0
Frappuccino®	9.5 fl. oz.	200	37	2 ½	6	3	2.0	15	100	0
Fruit 20®	8 fl. oz.	0	0	0	0	0	0.0	0	35	0
Fruit punch	8 fl. oz.	110	29	2	0	0	0.0	0	10	0
Gatorade®										
01 Prime	4 fl. oz.	100	25	1 ½	0	0	0.0	0	110	0
02 Perform	8 fl. oz.	50	14	1	0	0	0.0	0	110	0
02 Perform, low calorie	8 fl. oz.	20	5	0	0	0	0.0	0	110	0
03 Recover	8 fl. oz.	60	7	½	8	0	0.0	0	120	0
Hawaiian Punch®										
light	8 fl. oz.	10	2	0	0	0	0.0	0	120	0
regular	8 fl. oz.	80	21	1 ½	0	0	0.0	0	125	0
Hi-C®	8 fl. oz.	120	32	2	0	0	0.0	0	140	0
Hot cocoa										
sugar free, mix	8 fl. oz.	70	12	1	6	1	0.5	2	191	0
w/ 1% milk, hmde.	8 fl. oz.	175	24	1 ½	8	5	3.0	18	100	2
w/ water, mix	8 fl. oz.	120	23	1 ½	2	2	1.0	3	190	1
w/ whole milk, hmde.	8 fl. oz.	230	30	2	9	10	5.5	33	120	1
Kool-Aid®										
regular	8 fl. oz.	60	16	1	0	0	0.0	0	0	0
sugar free	8 fl. oz.	5	0	0	0	0	0.0	0	5	0

BEVERAGES

ITEM	AMOUNT	CALORIES	CARBOHYDRATE (g)	CARBOHYDRATE CHOICES	PROTEIN (g)	FAT (g)	SATURATED FAT (g)	CHOLESTEROL (mg)	SODIUM (mg)	FIBER (g)
Lemonade										
regular	8 fl. oz.	110	26	2	0	0	0.0	0	10	0
sugar free	8 fl. oz.	5	1	0	0	0	0.0	0	5	0
Quinine/tonic water	8 fl. oz.	83	22	1 ½	0	0	0.0	0	29	0
Red Bull® energy drink										
regular	8 fl. oz.	110	27	2	0	0	0.0	0	100	0
sugar free	8 fl. oz.	10	3	0	0	0	0.0	0	100	0
Rockstar® energy drink										
regular	8 fl. oz.	140	31	2	0	0	0.0	0	40	0
sugar free	8 fl. oz.	10	0	0	0	0	0.0	0	125	0
Soda, diet, most varieties	12 fl. oz.	0	0	0	0	0	0.0	0	35	0
Soda, regular										
7 Up®	12 fl. oz.	140	39	2 ½	0	0	0.0	0	40	0
Coca-Cola®/Coke®										
cherry	12 fl. oz.	150	42	3	0	0	0.0	0	35	0
regular	12 fl. oz.	140	39	2 ½	0	0	0.0	0	45	0
vanilla	12 fl. oz.	150	42	3	0	0	0.0	0	35	0
cream	12 fl. oz.	190	47	3	0	0	0.0	0	45	0
Dr. Pepper®	12 fl. oz.	150	40	2 ½	0	0	0.0	0	55	0
ginger ale	12 fl. oz.	120	33	2	0	0	0.0	0	38	0
grape	12 fl. oz.	190	48	3	0	0	0.0	0	45	0
Mello Yellow™	12 fl. oz.	170	47	3	0	0	0.0	0	45	0
Mountain Dew®	12 fl. oz.	170	46	3	0	0	0.0	0	65	0
Mountain Dew Code Red®	12 fl. oz.	170	46	3	0	0	0.0	0	105	0
Orange Crush®	12 fl. oz.	190	52	3 ½	0	0	0.0	0	70	0
Pepsi®										
regular	12 fl. oz.	150	41	3	0	0	0.0	0	30	0
wild cherry	12 fl. oz.	160	42	3	0	0	0.0	0	30	0
root beer	12 fl. oz.	170	42	3	0	0	0.0	0	45	0
Sierra Mist®	12 fl. oz.	140	37	2 ½	0	0	0.0	0	35	0
Sprite®	12 fl. oz.	140	38	2 ½	0	0	0.0	0	65	0
Squirt®	12 fl. oz.	140	39	2 ½	0	0	0.0	0	50	0
Tang®	8 fl. oz.	90	22	1 ½	0	0	0.0	0	35	0
Tea										
brewed/instant	6 fl. oz.	2	1	0	0	0	0.0	0	5	0
iced, diet, w/ lemon	8 fl. oz.	5	0	0	0	0	0.0	0	15	0
iced, sweetened	8 fl. oz.	80	22	1 ½	0	0	0.0	0	0	0
Vitamin Water®	8 fl. oz.	50	13	1	0	0	0.0	0	0	0
Water, bottled	8 fl. oz.	0	0	0	0	0	0.0	0	0	0
Yoo-hoo®	6.5 fl. oz.	100	24	1 ½	2	1	0.0	0	180	0

BREADS & BREAD PRODUCTS
Breads & Muffins

ITEM	AMOUNT	CALORIES	CARBOHYDRATE (g)	CARBOHYDRATE CHOICES	PROTEIN (g)	FAT (g)	SATURATED FAT (g)	CHOLESTEROL (mg)	SODIUM (mg)	FIBER (g)
BREADS & BREAD PRODUCTS										
Breads & Muffins										
Bagels										
blueberry										
medium	1 (2 oz.)	150	32	2	5	0	0.0	0	290	1
large	1 (5 oz.)	330	66	4 ½	10	3	0.5	0	600	2
cinnamon raisin										
medium	1 (2 oz.)	155	31	2	6	1	0.0	0	183	1
large	1 (5 oz.)	330	65	4	10	3	0.5	0	430	3
egg										
medium	1 (2 oz.)	158	30	2	6	1	0.0	14	286	1
large	1 (5 oz.)	315	60	4	12	2	0.5	27	573	3
plain										
mini	2 (0.9 oz.)	134	26	2	5	1	0.0	0	233	1
medium	1 (2 oz.)	150	31	2	5	0	0.0	0	313	1
large	1 (5 oz.)	320	62	4	12	3	0.5	0	650	2
Bialys	1 (4 inch)	138	32	2	7	0	0.0	0	333	1
Biscuits										
baking powder, can	1 (2 oz.)	190	24	1 ½	4	9	2.0	0	550	0
baking powder, hmde.	1 (2 oz.)	200	25	1 ½	4	9	2.5	2	329	1
buttermilk, can	1 (2 oz.)	170	26	2	4	6	3.5	0	590	0
buttermilk, hmde.	1 (2 oz.)	200	25	1 ½	4	9	2.5	2	329	1
Breads										
Boston brown, can	1 oz. slice	55	12	1	1	0	0.0	0	179	1
challah/egg	1 oz. slice	80	14	1	3	2	0.5	14	139	1
chapati	1 oz. slice	90	15	1	2	2	0.0	0	82	1
cracked wheat	1 oz. slice	74	14	1	2	1	0.5	0	153	2
French/Vienna	1 oz. slice	82	16	1	3	1	0.0	0	184	1
Ezekiel/sprouted	1.2 oz. slice	80	15	1	4	1	0.0	0	75	3
fruit	1 oz. slice	92	16	1	1	3	0.5	12	71	0
garlic	1 (2 inch)	170	13	1	3	12	2.5	0	240	0
Irish soda	1 oz. slice	82	16	1	2	1	0.5	5	113	1
Italian	1 oz. slice	77	14	1	2	1	0.0	0	166	1
low carb, multigrain	1 oz. slice	60	9	½	5	2	0.0	0	130	3
low carb, white	1 oz. slice	60	8	0	7	1	0.5	5	115	5
low protein	1 oz. slice	73	15	1	0	1	0.0	1	6	2
multigrain	1 oz. slice	71	13	1	3	1	0.0	0	138	2
oatmeal	1 oz. slice	76	14	1	2	1	0.0	0	170	1
pita, white	1 (6 inch)	165	33	2	5	1	0.0	0	322	1
pita, whole wheat	1 (6 inch)	170	35	2	6	2	0.5	0	340	5
pumpernickel	1 oz. slice	71	13	1	2	1	0.0	0	190	2
raisin	1 oz. slice	78	15	1	2	1	0.5	0	111	1

BREADS & BREAD PRODUCTS
Breads & Muffins

ITEM	AMOUNT	CALORIES	CARBOHYDRATE (g)	CARBOHYDRATE CHOICES	PROTEIN (g)	FAT (g)	SATURATED FAT (g)	CHOLESTEROL (mg)	SODIUM (mg)	FIBER (g)
Breads *(continued)*										
rye	1 oz. slice	73	14	1	2	1	0.0	0	187	2
sourdough	1 oz. slice	82	16	1	3	1	0.0	0	184	1
wheatberry	1 oz. slice	82	14	1	3	1	0.5	0	164	0
white	1 oz. slice	82	14	1	3	2	0.5	0	164	1
white, light	0.8 oz. slice	40	9	½	2	0	0.0	0	130	2
whole wheat	1 oz. slice	70	12	1	4	1	0.0	0	134	2
whole wheat, light	0.8 oz. slice	40	9	½	3	0	0.0	0	75	3
Breadsticks, soft	1 (2 oz.)	159	29	2	6	2	0.0	0	306	1
Cornbread	1 (2 oz.)	178	27	2	4	6	1.5	35	441	1
Croissants	1 (2 oz.)	230	26	2	5	12	6.5	38	422	1
English muffins										
plain	1 medium	129	25	1 ½	5	1	0.5	0	242	2
raisin	1 medium	137	27	2	5	1	0.5	0	189	1
whole wheat	1 medium	127	26	2	5	1	0.0	0	218	3
Melba toast	4	78	15	1	2	1	0.0	0	166	1
Muffins										
banana nut	1 (2 oz.)	190	29	2	3	7	1.5	5	370	1
blueberry	1 (2 oz.)	147	28	2	3	3	0.0	0	199	2
bran	1 (2 oz.)	153	27	2	4	4	0.5	0	223	3
chocolate chip	1 (2 oz.)	239	38	2 ½	3	10	3.5	21	113	1
corn	1 (2 oz.)	173	29	2	3	5	1.0	15	295	2
cranberry nut	1 (2 oz.)	157	27	2	3	4	0.5	17	253	1
lemon poppy seed	1 (2 oz.)	215	34	2	4	8	2.0	24	263	1
pumpkin	1 (2 oz.)	177	33	2	2	4	0.5	26	78	1
Popovers	1 (2 oz.)	146	14	1	5	8	3.5	97	116	0
Rolls										
brown & serve	1 medium	78	13	1	3	2	0.5	1	134	1
crescent	1 medium	110	11	1	2	6	1.5	0	220	0
French	1 medium	105	19	1	3	2	0.5	0	231	1
hamburger/hot dog	1 medium	120	21	1 ½	4	2	0.5	0	206	1
hard	1 medium	167	30	2	6	2	0.5	0	310	1
kaiser	1 medium	167	30	2	6	2	0.5	0	310	1
rye	1 medium	81	15	1	3	1	0.0	0	253	1
sesame seed	1 medium	140	23	1 ½	5	3	1.5	0	240	0
sourdough	1 medium	100	19	1	4	1	0.0	0	240	1
submarine	1 (8 inch)	220	44	3	7	2	0.0	0	460	2
whole wheat	1 medium	75	14	1	2	1	0.0	0	136	2
yeast	1 medium	106	18	1	3	3	0.5	0	126	0
Scones										
commercial	1 large	304	39	2 ½	8	13	4.0	100	345	1
hmde.	1 medium	150	19	1	4	6	2.0	49	171	1

BREADS & BREAD PRODUCTS
Bread Products

ITEM	AMOUNT	CALORIES	CARBOHYDRATE (g)	CARBOHYDRATE CHOICES	PROTEIN (g)	FAT (g)	SATURATED FAT (g)	CHOLESTEROL (mg)	SODIUM (mg)	FIBER (g)
Bread Products										
Corn fritters	1 (2 oz.)	117	14	1	3	6	2.0	5	279	1
Crêpes, plain	1 medium	30	5	0	1	1	0.0	5	50	0
Croutons	¼ cup	47	6	½	1	2	0.5	1	124	1
French toast										
frzn.	1 slice	126	19	1	4	4	1.0	48	292	1
hmde.	1 slice	149	16	1	5	7	2.0	75	311	1
Lefse	1 (2 oz.)	150	30	2	4	2	0.0	0	330	2
Pancakes										
blueberry, mix	2 (4 inch)	169	22	1 ½	5	7	1.5	43	313	1
buttermilk, mix	2 (4 inch)	173	22	1 ½	5	7	1.5	44	397	1
plain, frzn.	2 (4 inch)	122	24	1 ½	4	2	0.5	13	534	1
plain, hmde.	2 (4 inch)	173	22	1 ½	5	7	1.5	45	334	1
plain, lowfat, frzn.	2 (4 inch)	127	23	1 ½	4	1	0.5	20	253	1
whole wheat, mix	2 (4 inch)	183	26	2	7	6	1.5	54	503	2
Pizza crusts, Boboli®	1 (8 inch)	400	62	4	14	10	2.0	0	800	2
Pretzels, soft										
shopping mall type	1 large	391	83	5 ½	12	1	0.0	0	1035	3
Super Pretzel®, frzn.	1 medium	160	34	2	5	1	0.0	0	920	1
Stuffing										
bread, hmde.	½ cup	177	22	1 ½	3	9	1.5	0	543	3
cornbread, box	½ cup	179	22	1 ½	3	9	2.0	0	455	3
Stuffing, Stove Top®, box										
reduced sodium	½ cup	160	22	1 ½	3	7	1.5	0	330	0
regular	½ cup	160	21	1 ½	3	7	1.5	0	510	0
Taco shells, hard	1 (5 inch)	60	10	½	1	3	0.5	0	95	1
Tortillas										
corn	1 (6 inch)	57	12	1	1	1	0.0	0	12	2
flour	1 (8 inch)	146	25	1 ½	4	3	0.5	0	249	1
Waffles										
Belgian, mix	1 (7 inch)	370	59	4	10	10	2.0	0	1360	2
Blueberry Eggo®, frzn.	1 (1.3 oz.)	90	15	1	2	3	1.0	8	185	0
Homestyle Eggo®, frzn.	1 (1.3 oz.)	100	14	1	2	4	1.0	8	185	0
Nutrigrain Eggo®, frzn.	1 (1.3 oz.)	80	13	1	3	3	1.0	0	200	2
plain, frzn.	1 (1.3 oz.)	80	15	1	2	1	0.5	0	210	1
plain, hmde.	1 (7 inch)	218	25	1 ½	6	11	2.0	52	383	1
plain, lowfat, frzn.	1 (1.3 oz.)	83	15	1	2	1	0.5	9	155	0
CANDY										
Almonds										
candy-coated	10	165	24	1 ½	4	6	0.5	0	5	1
chocolate covered	10	175	15	1	4	13	4.0	4	17	3

CANDY

ITEM	AMOUNT	CALORIES	CARBOHYDRATE (g)	CARBOHYDRATE CHOICES	PROTEIN (g)	FAT (g)	SATURATED FAT (g)	CHOLESTEROL (mg)	SODIUM (mg)	FIBER (g)
Bit-o-Honey®	6 small	160	32	2	1	3	2.0	0	120	0
Bridge mix	¼ cup	190	26	2	2	8	4.5	5	40	0
Boston Baked Beans	11	70	11	1	1	2	0.0	0	0	1
Butterfinger® Minis	4	180	29	2	2	8	4.0	0	90	0
Cadbury Eggs®, creme	1 (1.4 oz.)	170	28	2	2	6	3.5	5	25	0
Candy bars, average size										
3 Musketeers®	1 (2.13 oz.)	260	46	3	2	8	5.0	5	110	1
5th Avenue®	1 (2.0 oz.)	260	38	2 ½	4	12	5.0	0	120	1
100 Grand®	1 (1.5 oz.)	190	30	2	1	8	5.0	5	90	0
Almond Joy®	1 (1.6 oz.)	220	26	2	2	13	8.0	0	50	2
Baby Ruth®	1 (2.1 oz.)	280	39	2 ½	4	14	8.0	0	130	1
Butterfinger®	1 (2.1 oz.)	270	43	3	4	11	6.0	0	135	1
Caramello®	1 (1.6 oz.)	220	29	2	3	10	6.0	10	45	0
Charleston Chew®	1 (1.4 oz.)	160	30	2	1	5	3.0	0	25	0
Chunky®	1 (1.4 oz.)	190	25	1 ½	2	11	5.0	5	15	1
Clark®	1 (2.10 oz.)	270	45	3	4	10	3.5	0	105	1
Heath Bar®	1 (1.4 oz.)	210	24	1 ½	1	13	7.0	10	135	0
Hershey's®, w/ almonds	1 (1.45 oz.)	210	21	1 ½	4	14	6.0	10	25	2
Hershey's® milk chocolate	1 (1.5 oz.)	210	26	2	3	13	8.0	10	35	1
Hershey's® special dark	1 (1.45 oz.)	180	25	1 ½	2	12	8.0	5	15	3
Kit Kat®	1 (1.5 oz.)	210	27	2	3	11	7.0	0	30	1
Milky Way®	1 (2.05 oz.)	270	41	3	2	11	7.0	5	95	1
Milky Way, Midnight®	1 (1.76 oz.)	230	36	2 ½	1	8	6.0	5	75	1
Mounds®	1 (1.75 oz.)	230	29	2	2	13	10.0	0	55	3
Mr. Goodbar®	1 (1.75 oz.)	250	26	2	5	17	7.0	0	65	2
Nestle's Crunch®	1 (1.55 oz.)	220	30	2	2	11	7.0	5	60	1
Oh Henry!®	1 (1.8 oz.)	240	32	2	4	10	5.0	0	120	0
Pay Day®	1 (1.85 oz.)	240	27	2	7	13	2.5	0	120	2
Pearson's® nut roll	1 (1.8 oz.)	240	27	2	4	11	2.0	0	170	2
Skor®	1 (1.4 oz.)	200	25	1 ½	1	12	7.0	20	130	0
Snickers®	1 (2.07 oz.)	280	35	2	4	14	5.0	5	140	1
Symphony®	1 (1.35 oz.)	200	22	1 ½	3	12	7.0	10	40	1
Twix®	1 (1.79 oz.)	250	33	2	2	12	9.0	5	100	1
Whatchamacallit®	1 (1.6 oz.)	230	28	2	3	12	9.0	0	140	0
Candy corn	22	140	36	2 ½	0	0	0.0	0	115	0
Caramels	6	183	37	2 ½	2	4	3.0	3	118	1
Cherries, chocolate covered	2	110	18	1	1	4	2.5	0	15	2
Circus peanuts	6	160	39	2 ½	0	0	0.0	0	0	0
Cotton candy	1 oz.	113	28	2	0	0	0.0	0	0	0
Divinity, hmde.	2 (0.4 oz.)	83	20	1	0	0	0.0	0	8	0
Dots®	11	130	33	2	0	0	0.0	0	15	0
Ferrero Rocher®	3	220	16	1	3	16	5.0	0	15	1

CANDY

ITEM	AMOUNT	CALORIES	CARBOHYDRATE (g)	CARBOHYDRATE CHOICES	PROTEIN (g)	FAT (g)	SATURATED FAT (g)	CHOLESTEROL (mg)	SODIUM (mg)	FIBER (g)
Fondant	2 (0.5 oz.)	106	26	2	0	0	0.0	0	5	0
Fudge, hmde.										
chocolate, w/ nuts	1 oz.	131	19	1	1	5	1.5	3	12	1
chocolate, w/o nuts	1 oz.	117	22	1 ½	1	3	1.5	4	13	0
vanilla, w/ nuts	1 oz.	123	21	1 ½	1	4	1.0	4	13	0
vanilla, w/o nuts	1 oz.	109	23	1 ½	0	2	1.0	4	14	0
Ghirardelli® Chocolate Squares™										
dark	4 squares	210	23	1 ½	2	16	10.0	0	0	3
milk	4 squares	220	25	1 ½	3	14	9.0	10	30	0
milk, w/ caramel	3 squares	220	27	2	2	12	7.0	10	60	0
Goobers®	¼ cup	210	22	1 ½	5	14	5.0	5	15	2
Good & Fruity™	43	150	37	2 ½	0	0	0.0	0	25	0
Good & Plenty®	33	140	35	2	0	0	0.0	0	120	0
Gum, regular/sugar free	1 stick	7	2	0	0	0	0.0	0	0	0
Gumdrops	10	143	36	2 ½	0	0	0.0	0	16	0
Gummy bears	15	131	33	2	0	0	0.0	0	15	0
Hard candies										
regular	3 small	35	9	½	0	0	0.0	0	3	0
sugar free	3 small	34	8	½	0	0	0.0	0	0	0
Hershey's Hugs®	9	210	24	1 ½	3	12	7.0	10	45	0
Hershey's Kisses®	9	200	25	1 ½	3	12	7.0	10	35	1
Hershey's Kisses®, w/ almonds	9	210	21	1 ½	4	14	7.0	10	30	1
Hot Tamales®	20	150	36	2 ½	0	0	0.0	0	15	0
Jelly beans	35 small	140	37	2 ½	0	0	0.0	0	15	0
Jolly Rancher®	3	70	17	1	0	0	0.0	0	0	0
Junior® mints	16	170	35	2	1	3	2.5	0	30	1
Licorice, black/red	3 (8 inch)	120	27	2	1	1	0.0	0	85	0
Lifesavers®	4	45	11	1	0	0	0.0	0	0	0
Lollipops										
Blow Pop®	1	60	17	1	0	0	0.0	0	0	0
Dum Dums®	1	26	7	½	0	0	0.0	0	0	0
Saf-T-Pop®	1	43	11	1	0	0	0.0	0	0	0
Tootsie Pop®	1	60	15	1	0	0	0.0	0	0	0
M&M's®										
crispy	52	200	31	2	2	8	5.0	5	60	1
peanut	18	250	30	2	5	13	5.0	5	25	2
plain	52	240	34	2	2	10	6.0	5	30	1
Malted milk balls	10	180	32	2	1	6	5.0	0	75	0
Marshmallows	4 large	90	23	1 ½	0	0	0.0	0	30	0
Mary Janes®	5	160	32	2	1	4	0.5	0	65	0
Mike and Ike®	23	140	36	2 ½	0	0	0.0	0	25	0
Milk Duds®	13	170	28	2	1	6	3.5	0	100	0

CANDY

ITEM	AMOUNT	CALORIES	CARBOHYDRATE (g)	CARBOHYDRATE CHOICES	PROTEIN (g)	FAT (g)	SATURATED FAT (g)	CHOLESTEROL (mg)	SODIUM (mg)	FIBER (g)
Mints										
Altoids®	3	10	2	0	0	0	0.0	0	0	0
Breath Savers®	1	5	2	0	0	0	0.0	0	0	0
butter	6	51	12	1	0	0	0.0	0	21	0
Nips®, caramel	2	60	11	1	0	2	1.5	0	40	0
Nonpareils	12	230	35	2	2	11	6.0	0	0	0
Orange slices	3	150	38	2 ½	0	0	0.0	0	15	0
Peanut brittle	½ cup	180	30	2	4	5	1.0	0	130	1
Peanuts, chocolate covered	¼ cup	193	18	1	5	12	5.5	3	15	2
Peeps®	3	110	28	2	1	0	0.0	0	10	0
Pez®	12	35	9	½	0	0	0.0	0	0	0
Praline, hmde.	1 (1.4 oz.)	173	22	1 ½	1	10	3.0	10	40	1
Raisinets®	¼ cup	190	32	2	2	8	5.0	5	15	1
Raisins, yogurt covered	¼ cup	188	35	2	2	6	5.0	0	21	1
Red Raspberry Dollars®	10	120	31	2	0	0	0.0	0	20	0
Reese's Peanut Butter Cups®	2 (0.8 oz.)	210	24	1 ½	5	13	4.5	0	150	1
Reese's Pieces®	51	190	25	1 ½	4	9	7.0	0	75	1
Rolo®	7	190	29	2	2	9	6.0	5	70	0
Skittles®	¼ cup	170	39	2 ½	0	2	2.0	0	5	0
Sour Patch Kids®	16	140	36	2 ½	0	0	0.0	0	25	0
Starburst®	8	160	34	2	0	3	3.0	0	0	0
Sugar Babies®	30	180	41	3	0	2	0.0	0	40	0
Sugar Daddy®	1 (1.7 oz.)	200	43	3	1	3	0.5	0	65	0
Swedish Fish®										
small	26 (1 inch)	200	51	3 ½	0	0	0.0	0	40	0
medium	7 (2 inch)	150	38	2 ½	0	0	0.0	0	30	0
Sweet Escapes, Hershey's®										
caramel fudge bar	1 (0.7 oz.)	80	14	1	0	2	1.0	0	55	0
chocolate wafer bar	1 (0.7 oz.)	80	14	1	1	3	1.5	0	30	0
peanut butter bar	1 (0.7 oz.)	90	13	1	2	3	2.0	0	50	0
Sweet Tarts®	8 small	60	14	1	0	0	0.0	0	0	0
Taffy										
Air Heads®	1 (4 inch)	60	14	1	0	1	0.5	0	8	0
saltwater	8 small	150	36	2 ½	0	1	1.0	0	10	0
Tic Tac®	1	2	0	0	0	0	0.0	0	0	0
Toblerone®	4 triangles	170	21	1 ½	2	10	6.0	5	20	0
Tootsie Roll®	6 small	140	28	2	1	3	0.5	0	15	0
Truffles	1 (0.4 oz.)	73	5	0	1	6	4.0	2	7	0
Turtles	2 (0.6 oz.)	160	20	1	2	9	3.0	5	40	0
Whoppers®	18	180	31	2	1	7	7.0	0	115	0
York Peppermint Pattie®	1 (1.4 oz.)	140	31	2	0	3	1.5	0	10	0

CEREAL BARS & CEREALS
Cereal Bars

ITEM	AMOUNT	CALORIES	CARBOHYDRATE (g)	CARBOHYDRATE CHOICES	PROTEIN (g)	FAT (g)	SATURATED FAT (g)	CHOLESTEROL (mg)	SODIUM (mg)	FIBER (g)
CEREAL BARS & CEREALS										
Cereal Bars										
Balance Bar®	1 bar	200	21	1 ½	15	7	3.0	0	170	0
Clif Bar®	1 bar	250	42	2 ½	11	6	1.0	0	230	5
Crunchy granola										
cinnamon	1 bar	90	15	1	2	3	0.0	0	80	1
maple brown sugar	1 bar	90	15	1	2	3	0.0	0	80	1
oats 'n honey	1 bar	90	15	1	2	3	0.0	0	80	1
peanut butter	1 bar	90	15	1	2	4	0.0	0	95	1
Fiber One®	1 bar	140	30	1 ½	2	3	0.5	0	90	9
Fiber Plus™ antioxidants	1 bar	130	24	1	2	5	2.5	0	50	9
Fruit & oatmeal										
apple crisp	1 bar	130	26	2	1	3	0.5	0	85	1
strawberry crisp	1 bar	130	26	2	1	3	0.5	0	100	1
Kashi® GoLean® Crunchy!										
chocolate almond	1 bar	170	27	1 ½	8	5	2.5	0	210	5
chocolate caramel	1 bar	150	28	1 ½	8	3	2.0	0	220	6
chocolate peanut	1 bar	180	30	2	9	5	2.0	0	250	6
Milk & cereal										
Cinnamon Toast Crunch®	1 bar	180	33	2	3	4	2.0	0	150	1
Honey Nut Cheerios®	1 bar	160	28	2	3	4	2.0	0	90	1
Nutri-Grain®										
apple cinnamon	1 bar	120	24	1 ½	2	3	0.5	0	110	3
blueberry	1 bar	120	24	1 ½	2	3	0.5	0	110	3
strawberry	1 bar	120	24	1 ½	2	3	0.5	0	110	3
Nutri-Grain®, SuperFruit Fusion™										
cherry pomegranate	1 bar	130	25	1 ½	2	3	0.5	0	85	3
strawberry acai	1 bar	130	26	2	2	4	0.5	0	105	3
Power Bar®										
harvest energy	1 bar	240	42	2 ½	10	4	0.5	0	140	5
performance	1 bar	240	45	3	8	4	0.5	0	200	1
Quaker Chewy® granola										
25% less sugar	1 bar	100	17	1	1	2	0.5	0	80	1
chocolate chip	1 bar	100	17	1	1	3	1.0	0	75	1
chocolate swirl	1 bar	90	18	1	1	2	0.5	0	80	1
peanut butter, chocolate chip	1 bar	100	17	1	2	3	1.0	0	95	1
Rice Krispies Treats®	1 bar	90	17	1	0	3	1.0	0	105	0
South Beach Living	1 bar	140	17	1	8	5	2.0	0	120	3
Special K®										
blueberry	1 bar	90	18	1	0	2	1.0	0	85	3
strawberry	1 bar	90	18	1	0	2	1.0	0	85	3
Special K®, fruit crisps	1 bar	50	10	½	1	1	0.5	0	40	0

CEREAL BARS & CEREALS

Cooked Cereals, prepared with water

ITEM	AMOUNT	CALORIES	CARBOHYDRATE (g)	CARBOHYDRATE CHOICES	PROTEIN (g)	FAT (g)	SATURATED FAT (g)	CHOLESTEROL (mg)	SODIUM (mg)	FIBER (g)
Cooked Cereals, prepared w/ water										
Cream of Rice®	1 cup	170	36	2 ½	3	0	0.0	0	0	0
Cream of Wheat®	1 cup	120	24	1 ½	4	0	0.0	0	0	1
Grits, corn										
instant	1 pkt.	100	22	1 ½	2	0	0.0	0	310	1
old fashioned	1 cup	150	32	2	4	1	0.0	0	0	1
quick	1 cup	130	29	2	3	1	0.0	0	0	2
Maltex®	1 cup	180	38	2	5	1	0.0	0	0	5
Malt-O-Meal®	1 cup	130	27	2	5	1	0.0	0	0	1
Maypo®	1 cup	180	34	2	5	3	0.5	0	105	4
Oat bran	1 cup	130	25	1 ½	7	3	0.5	0	0	6
Oatmeal										
apples & cinnamon, instant	1 pkt.	130	27	2	3	2	0.5	0	160	3
cinnamon & spice, instant	1 pkt.	160	32	2	4	3	0.5	0	210	3
maple & brown sugar, instant	1 pkt.	160	32	2	4	3	0.5	0	260	3
peaches & cream, instant	1 pkt.	130	27	2	3	2	0.5	0	180	2
raisins & spice, instant	1 pkt.	150	32	2	4	2	0.0	0	210	3
regular, instant	1 pkt.	100	19	1	4	2	0.0	0	75	3
regular, old fashioned/quick	1 cup	150	27	2	5	3	0.5	0	0	4
steel cut	1 cup	150	27	2	5	3	0.5	0	0	4
Wheatena®	1 cup	160	32	2	5	1	0.0	0	0	5
Ready To Eat Cereals										
All-Bran®										
bran buds	½ cup	70	24	1	2	1	0.0	0	200	13
original	½ cup	80	23	1	4	1	0.0	0	80	10
Alpha-Bits®	1 cup	110	23	1 ½	2	1	0.0	0	180	2
Amaranth flakes	1 cup	140	26	2	4	2	0.0	0	120	3
Apple Jacks®	1 cup	100	25	1 ½	1	1	0.0	0	130	3
Banana Nut Crunch®	1 cup	240	44	3	5	6	0.5	0	230	4
Basic 4®	1 cup	200	44	3	4	3	1.0	0	290	4
Blueberry Morning®	1¼ cups	220	45	3	3	3	0.0	0	260	2
Bran flakes	¾ cup	90	23	1	3	1	0.0	0	210	5
Cap'n Crunch®										
Crunch Berries®	¾ cup	100	22	1 ½	1	2	1.0	0	190	1
original	¾ cup	110	23	1 ½	1	2	1.0	0	200	1
Peanut Butter Crunch®	¾ cup	110	21	1 ½	2	3	1.0	0	200	1
Cheerios®										
apple cinnamon	¾ cup	120	24	1 ½	2	2	0.0	0	135	2
banana nut	¾ cup	100	24	1 ½	1	1	0.0	0	160	2
frosted	¾ cup	110	23	1 ½	2	1	0.0	0	170	2
honey nut	¾ cup	110	22	1 ½	2	2	0.0	0	160	2

CEREAL BARS & CEREALS
Ready to Eat Cereals

ITEM	AMOUNT	CALORIES	CARBOHYDRATE (g)	CARBOHYDRATE CHOICES	PROTEIN (g)	FAT (g)	SATURATED FAT (g)	CHOLESTEROL (mg)	SODIUM (mg)	FIBER (g)
Cheerios® *(continued)*										
multi-grain	1 cup	110	23	1 ½	2	1	0.0	0	160	3
original	1 cup	100	20	1	3	2	0.0	0	160	3
Yogurt Burst®, vanilla	¾ cup	120	24	1 ½	2	2	0.5	0	180	2
Chex®										
cinnamon	¾ cup	120	25	1 ½	1	2	0.0	0	180	0
corn	1 cup	120	26	2	2	1	0.0	0	240	1
multi-bran	¾ cup	160	39	2 ½	4	2	0.0	0	270	6
rice	1 cup	100	23	1 ½	2	1	0.0	0	240	1
wheat	¾ cup	160	39	2 ½	5	1	0.0	0	300	5
Cinnamon Toast Crunch®	¾ cup	130	25	1 ½	1	3	0.5	0	220	1
Cocoa Pebbles®	¾ cup	120	26	2	1	2	1.0	0	190	0
Cocoa Puffs®	¾ cup	110	22	1 ½	1	2	0.0	0	150	2
Cocoa Rice Krispies®	¾ cup	120	27	2	1	1	0.5	0	130	0
Cookie Crisp®	¾ cup	100	22	1 ½	1	1	0.0	0	150	1
Corn Flakes®	1 cup	100	24	1 ½	2	0	0.0	0	200	1
Corn Pops®	1 cup	120	29	2	1	0	0.0	0	125	3
Cracklin' Oat Bran®	¾ cup	200	35	2	4	7	3.0	0	150	6
Cranberry Almond Crunch®	¾ cup	200	40	2 ½	4	3	0.0	0	115	3
Crispix®	1 cup	110	25	1 ½	2	0	0.0	0	220	0
Crunchy oatmeal squares	1 cup	210	44	3	6	3	0.5	0	250	5
Fiber One®										
honey clusters	½ cup	160	25	1	3	2	0.0	0	230	13
original	½ cup	60	25	1	2	1	0.0	0	105	14
raisin bran clusters	1 cup	170	47	3	3	1	0.0	0	210	11
Flax Plus®, organic										
maple pecan crunch	¾ cup	220	38	2	6	7	1.0	0	190	5
multibran	¾ cup	110	23	1	4	2	0.0	0	135	5
Froot Loops®	1 cup	110	25	1 ½	1	1	0.5	0	135	3
Frosted Flakes®	¾ cup	110	27	2	1	0	0.0	0	140	1
Fruity Pebbles®	¾ cup	120	26	2	1	1	1.0	0	190	0
Golden Crisp®	¾ cup	110	24	1 ½	2	0	0.0	0	25	0
Golden Grahams®	¾ cup	120	26	2	2	1	0.0	0	270	1
Granola										
lowfat	½ cup	190	39	2 ½	4	3	0.5	0	120	3
lowfat, w/ raisins	½ cup	170	36	2 ½	4	2	0.0	0	115	2
regular	½ cup	220	32	2	5	9	4.0	0	25	4
regular, w/ raisins	½ cup	220	35	2	5	8	3.5	0	25	3
Grape-nuts®										
flakes	¾ cup	110	24	1 ½	3	1	0.0	0	125	3
original	½ cup	200	48	3	6	1	0.0	0	290	7

CEREAL BARS & CEREALS
Ready to Eat Cereals

ITEM	AMOUNT	CALORIES	CARBOHYDRATE (g)	CARBOHYDRATE CHOICES	PROTEIN (g)	FAT (g)	SATURATED FAT (g)	CHOLESTEROL (mg)	SODIUM (mg)	FIBER (g)
Great Grains®										
crunchy pecans	¾ cup	210	37	2	5	6	0.5	0	160	5
raisins, dates & pecans	¾ cup	200	40	2 ½	4	4	0.0	0	160	5
Honey Bunches of Oats®										
original	¾ cup	120	25	1 ½	2	2	0.0	0	150	2
w/ almonds	¾ cup	130	25	1 ½	2	3	0.0	0	140	2
Honey Smacks®	¾ cup	100	24	1 ½	2	1	0.0	0	50	1
Honeycomb®	1½ cups	130	28	2	2	1	0.0	0	180	1
Kashi®										
GoLean®	1 cup	140	30	1 ½	13	1	0.0	0	85	10
GoLean Crunch!®	1 cup	190	37	2	9	3	0.0	0	100	8
GoLean Crunch!®, honey almond flax	1 cup	200	36	2	9	5	0.0	0	140	8
Good Friends®	1 cup	160	42	2 ½	5	2	0.0	0	110	12
Good Friends®, cinna-raisin	1 cup	170	41	2 ½	4	2	0.0	0	105	8
Heart to Heart®, blueberry clusters	1 cup	200	44	3	6	2	0.0	0	135	4
Heart to Heart®, honey toasted	¾ cup	120	25	1 ½	4	2	0.0	0	85	5
Heart to Heart®, warm cinnamon	¾ cup	120	25	1 ½	4	2	0.0	0	80	5
honey puffs	1 cup	120	25	1 ½	3	1	0.0	0	5	2
Kix®										
berry berry	¾ cup	100	22	1 ½	1	1	0.0	0	180	1
original	1¼ cups	110	25	1 ½	2	1	0.0	0	190	3
Life®	¾ cup	120	25	1 ½	3	2	0.0	0	160	2
Lucky Charms®	¾ cup	110	22	1 ½	2	1	0.0	0	190	1
Mini-Wheats®										
frosted, big bite	5 biscuits	180	41	2 ½	5	1	0.0	0	5	5
frosted, bite size	24 biscuits	200	48	3	6	1	0.0	0	5	6
Mueslix®	⅔ cup	200	40	2 ½	5	3	0.0	0	170	4
Oat bran flakes	¾ cup	110	23	1 ½	3	1	0.0	0	210	4
Oatmeal Squares	1 cup	210	44	3	6	3	0.5	0	190	5
Product 19®	1 cup	100	25	1 ½	2	0	0.0	0	210	1
Puffed rice	1 cup	70	15	1	1	0	0.0	0	0	0
Puffed wheat	1 cup	60	13	1	3	0	0.0	0	0	2
Raisin bran	1 cup	190	46	3	5	1	0.0	0	320	7
Raisin Bran Crunch®	1 cup	190	45	3	3	1	0.0	0	210	4
Reese's® Puffs®	¾ cup	120	22	1 ½	2	3	0.5	0	180	1
Rice Krispies®	1¼ cups	130	29	2	2	0	0.0	0	190	0
Shredded Wheat®										
frosted, Spoon Size®	1 cup	180	44	3	4	1	0.0	0	0	5
honey nut	1 cup	190	44	3	4	2	0.0	0	70	5
original	2 biscuits	160	37	2	5	1	0.0	0	0	6
original, Spoon Size®	1 cup	170	40	2 ½	6	1	0.0	0	0	6
Wheat 'N Bran, Spoon Size®	1¼ cups	200	49	3	6	1	0.0	0	0	8

CEREAL BARS & CEREALS
Ready to Eat Cereals

ITEM	AMOUNT	CALORIES	CARBOHYDRATE (g)	CARBOHYDRATE CHOICES	PROTEIN (g)	FAT (g)	SATURATED FAT (g)	CHOLESTEROL (mg)	SODIUM (mg)	FIBER (g)
Smart Start®, strong heart	1 cup	190	43	3	3	1	0.0	0	280	3
Special K®										
fruit & yogurt	¾ cup	120	27	2	2	1	0.0	0	135	3
original	1 cup	120	23	1 ½	6	1	0.0	0	220	0
red berries	1 cup	110	27	2	2	0	0.0	0	190	3
Total®										
blueberry pomegranate	1 cup	170	38	2 ½	5	2	0.0	0	95	4
cinnamon crunch	1 cup	190	40	2 ½	4	3	0.0	0	200	4
raisin bran	1 cup	160	40	2 ½	3	1	0.0	0	230	5
whole grain	¾ cup	100	23	1 ½	2	1	0.0	0	190	3
Trix®	1 cup	120	28	2	1	2	0.0	0	190	1
Weetabix®	2 biscuits	130	29	2	4	1	0.0	0	130	4
Wheat bran flakes	¾ cup	90	23	1	3	1	0.0	0	210	5
Wheat flakes	1 cup	120	25	1 ½	3	1	0.0	0	125	3
Wheat germ	2 T.	50	6	½	3	1	0.0	0	0	2
Wheaties®	¾ cup	100	22	1 ½	3	1	0.0	0	190	3

CHEESE
ITEM	AMOUNT	CALORIES	CARBOHYDRATE (g)	CARBOHYDRATE CHOICES	PROTEIN (g)	FAT (g)	SATURATED FAT (g)	CHOLESTEROL (mg)	SODIUM (mg)	FIBER (g)
American										
fat free	1 oz.	41	3	0	7	0	0.0	7	364	0
reduced fat	1 oz.	51	1	0	7	2	1.5	10	405	0
regular	1 oz.	106	0	0	6	9	5.5	27	422	0
American, singles										
fat free	1 slice	30	2	0	5	0	0.0	3	276	0
reduced fat	1 slice	45	1	0	4	3	1.5	10	260	0
regular	1 slice	60	2	0	3	5	2.5	15	240	0
Blue	1 oz.	100	1	0	6	8	5.0	25	390	0
Brick	1 oz.	105	1	0	7	8	5.5	27	159	0
Brie	1 oz.	95	0	0	6	8	5.0	28	178	0
Camembert	1 oz.	85	0	0	6	7	4.5	20	239	0
Caraway	1 oz.	107	1	0	7	8	5.5	26	196	0
Cheddar										
fat free	1 oz.	40	1	0	8	0	0.0	3.0	220	0
reduced fat	1 oz.	70	1	0	8	5	3.0	15	170	0
regular	1 oz.	40	1	0	8	0	0.0	3	220	0
regular, shredded	¼ cup	114	0	0	7	9	6.0	30	176	0
spread	2 T.	80	1	0	4	7	4.5	22	461	0
Cheez Whiz®	2 T.	90	4	0	3	7	1.5	5	440	0
Colby	1 oz.	111	1	0	7	9	6.0	30	182	0
Colby & Monterey Jack	1 oz.	111	0	0	7	9	6.0	30	182	0
Cottage										
1% fat	½ cup	81	3	0	14	1	0.5	5	459	0

CHEESE

ITEM	AMOUNT	CALORIES	CARBOHYDRATE (g)	CARBOHYDRATE CHOICES	PROTEIN (g)	FAT (g)	SATURATED FAT (g)	CHOLESTEROL (mg)	SODIUM (mg)	FIBER (g)
Cottage *(continued)*										
2% fat	½ cup	102	4	0	16	2	1.5	9	459	0
fat free	½ cup	80	8	½	12	0	0.0	10	460	0
Cream										
fat free	2 T.	30	2	0	5	0	0.0	5	200	0
light	2 T.	70	2	0	3	5	3.5	15	150	0
regular	2 T.	101	1	0	2	10	6.5	32	86	0
Cream, flavored										
onion & chive, light	2 T.	60	3	0	2	5	3.0	15	170	0
onion & chive, regular	2 T.	90	2	0	2	9	5.0	35	160	0
strawberry, regular	2 T.	90	5	0	1	8	4.5	30	120	0
Easy Cheese®, cheddar	2 T.	90	2	0	5	6	3.0	20	410	0
Edam	1 oz.	101	0	0	7	8	5.0	25	274	0
Feta	1 oz.	60	1	0	5	5	3.0	10	350	0
Fondue	¼ cup	123	2	0	8	7	4.5	24	71	0
Fontina	1 oz.	101	0	0	6	8	4.0	25	172	0
Goat, soft	1 oz.	76	0	0	5	6	4.0	13	104	0
Gorgonzola	1 oz.	101	0	0	6	8	5.0	30	283	0
Gouda	1 oz.	101	1	0	7	8	5.0	32	232	0
Gruyere	1 oz.	117	0	0	8	9	5.5	31	95	0
Havarti	1 oz.	111	0	0	7	9	6.0	25	172	0
Jarlsberg	1 oz.	95	1	0	7	7	4.0	18	130	0
Limburger	1 oz.	93	0	0	6	8	4.5	26	227	0
Mascarpone	1 oz.	122	0	0	2	13	7.0	35	15	0
Monterey Jack	1 oz.	101	0	0	6	9	5.0	30	192	0
Mozzarella										
part-skim	1 oz.	81	1	0	7	6	3.5	15	192	0
whole milk	1 oz.	91	1	0	7	7	5.0	25	192	0
Muenster	1 oz.	104	0	0	7	9	5.5	27	178	0
Neufchatel	1 oz.	74	1	0	3	7	4.0	22	113	0
Parmesan										
grated	1 T.	30	0	0	3	2	1.5	8	128	0
grated, reduced fat	1 T.	20	2	0	1	1	0.5	5	80	0
hard, shredded	1 T.	30	0	0	3	2	1.0	5	125	0
Pepper Jack	1 oz.	111	1	0	6	9	5.0	30	172	0
Port wine, cold pack										
light	2 T.	70	5	0	5	4	2.0	15	190	0
regular	2 T.	90	3	0	5	7	3.0	20	210	0
Provolone	1 oz.	100	1	0	7	8	5.0	20	248	0
Ricotta										
fat free	½ cup	100	10	½	10	0	0.0	20	130	0
lowfat	½ cup	120	6	½	10	5	3.0	30	110	0

CHEESE

ITEM	AMOUNT	CALORIES	CARBOHYDRATE (g)	CARBOHYDRATE CHOICES	PROTEIN (g)	FAT (g)	SATURATED FAT (g)	CHOLESTEROL (mg)	SODIUM (mg)	FIBER (g)
Ricotta *(continued)*										
part-skim	½ cup	140	6	½	12	9	6.0	50	170	0
whole milk	½ cup	180	6	½	14	12	8.0	50	150	0
Romano, grated	1 T.	30	0	0	3	2	1.5	8	128	0
Roquefort	1 oz.	105	1	0	6	9	5.5	26	513	0
Soy cheese	1 oz.	50	0	0	6	3	0.0	0	411	0
String	1 oz.	83	1	0	7	5	3.5	18	236	0
Swiss										
natural	1 oz.	110	1	0	9	8	5.0	30	60	0
processed	1 oz.	91	1	0	6	7	4.5	25	344	0
Velveeta®	1 oz.	80	3	0	5	6	3.5	20	370	0
Yogurt cheese	1 oz.	22	3	0	2	0	0.0	1	22	0

COMBINATION FOODS, FROZEN ENTRÉES & MEALS

ITEM	AMOUNT	CALORIES	CARBOHYDRATE (g)	CARBOHYDRATE CHOICES	PROTEIN (g)	FAT (g)	SATURATED FAT (g)	CHOLESTEROL (mg)	SODIUM (mg)	FIBER (g)
Bagel Bites®, frzn.										
cheese & pepperoni	4 pieces	190	29	2	8	6	2.5	15	380	2
mozzarella	4 pieces	190	26	2	8	5	3.0	15	380	2
three cheese	4 pieces	190	28	2	7	5	2.5	10	370	2
Baked beans, w/ pork, can	½ cup	150	29	1 ½	7	1	0.0	0	550	7
Beans & rice, box	1 cup	190	40	2 ½	8	0	0.0	0	720	5
Beef goulash, w/ noodles	1 cup	361	27	2	30	14	3.5	95	130	2
Beef Oriental	1 cup	104	12	1	10	2	0.5	12	969	4
Beef stroganoff, w/ noodles	1 cup	344	23	1 ½	20	19	7.5	74	468	2
Beefaroni®, can	1 cup	240	30	2	9	9	3.5	15	720	3
Burritos, frzn.										
bean & cheese	1 (6 oz.)	413	66	4	13	11	2.5	5	941	6
beef & bean	1 (6 oz.)	352	51	3	11	11	4.0	9	866	6
chicken & black bean	1 (6 oz.)	282	32	2	13	13	5.0	25	409	4
Casseroles										
chicken, w/ cheese sauce	1 cup	368	9	½	44	16	6.5	136	739	0
green bean	1 cup	300	22	1 ½	6	20	6.0	10	1240	4
seafood Newburg	1 cup	613	10	½	30	50	29.5	426	551	0
tuna noodle	1 cup	238	25	1 ½	17	7	2.0	41	686	1
Chicken cacciatore w/ pasta	1 cup	320	9	½	29	18	4.5	89	172	1
Chicken cordon bleu	6 oz.	281	27	2	15	13	4.0	35	886	3
Chicken divan	6 oz.	249	10	½	16	16	7.0	61	479	1
Chicken Helper®, box										
creamy chicken & noodles	1 cup	280	24	1 ½	25	9	2.5	60	750	0
fettucini Alfredo	1 cup	280	27	2	25	7	2.5	55	790	1
Chicken nuggets, frzn.	4 pieces	210	9	½	11	15	3.5	35	360	1
Chicken parmigiana, frzn.	1 (6 oz.)	202	18	1	6	11	4.0	32	570	2
Chicken tetrazzini	1 cup	366	28	2	19	19	7.0	49	705	2

COMBINATION FOODS, FROZEN ENTRÉES & MEALS

ITEM	AMOUNT	CALORIES	CARBOHYDRATE (g)	CARBOHYDRATE CHOICES	PROTEIN (g)	FAT (g)	SATURATED FAT (g)	CHOLESTEROL (mg)	SODIUM (mg)	FIBER (g)
Chili, w/ beans, can										
beef	1 cup	247	34	2	16	7	3.0	30	1220	7
turkey	1 cup	247	26	1 ½	17	3	1.0	45	1200	5
Chimichangas, frzn.										
beef	1 (4.5 oz.)	360	37	2 ½	9	20	5.0	10	470	3
chicken	1 (4.5 oz.)	340	39	2 ½	11	16	4.0	20	540	2
Chipped beef, creamed	1 (6 oz.)	187	12	1	13	10	6.0	43	801	1
Chop suey, can										
beef	1 cup	271	12	1	22	15	3.5	50	924	3
chicken	1 cup	193	10	½	20	8	1.5	50	651	2
pork	1 cup	286	12	1	22	17	4.0	56	926	3
Chow mein, can										
beef	1 cup	271	12	1	22	15	3.5	50	924	3
chicken	1 cup	193	10	½	20	8	1.5	50	651	2
Corn dogs, frzn.	1 (2.7 oz.)	220	22	1 ½	6	12	3.5	25	540	0
Easy Express® skillets										
chicken & vegetables	½ pkg.	360	43	3	26	9	2.5	40	860	4
chicken Alfredo	½ pkg.	410	48	3	31	10	4.0	50	980	6
garlic shrimp	½ pkg.	310	40	2 ½	15	10	2.0	50	1110	5
yankee pot roast	½ pkg.	300	38	2 ½	18	8	3.0	40	930	4
Egg rolls										
pork	1 (6 oz.)	220	24	1 ½	5	11	2.5	10	390	2
shrimp	1 (6 oz.)	180	25	1 ½	5	7	1.5	15	490	2
Eggplant parmigiana	1 cup	440	38	2	10	28	8.0	20	1060	6
Enchiladas										
beef & cheese	1 (6 oz.)	286	27	2	11	16	8.0	36	1169	3
chicken	1 (6 oz.)	193	28	2	10	5	1.5	13	374	3
Fajitas										
beef	1 (6 oz.)	305	27	2	17	14	4.0	34	241	2
chicken	1 (6 oz.)	277	34	2	15	9	1.5	30	262	4
Frozen breakfasts										
cinnamon French toast, w/ sausage	1 (5.5 oz.)	415	38	2 ½	13	23	7.5	98	502	2
egg, steak & cheese bagel	1 (4.5 oz.)	360	29	2	20	18	7.0	166	676	0
pancakes, w/ sausage	1 (6 oz.)	490	52	3 ½	14	25	11.0	90	951	3
sausage, egg & cheese biscuit	1 (4.2 oz.)	351	28	2	12	21	8.5	88	809	2
scrambled eggs & bacon	1 (5.3 oz.)	292	17	1	11	19	9.0	242	706	1
scrambled eggs & sausage, w/ hashed browns	1 (6.3 oz.)	364	17	1	13	27	7.5	286	779	1
Frozen dinners										
beef tips, w/ mushroom sauce	1 (14 oz.)	443	40	2 ½	26	20	7.0	51	1667	6
chicken, BBQ, w/ potatoes & corn	1 (10 oz.)	267	43	3	14	4	0.5	29	605	4

COMBINATION FOODS, FROZEN ENTRÉES & MEALS

ITEM	AMOUNT	CALORIES	CARBOHYDRATE (g)	CARBOHYDRATE CHOICES	PROTEIN (g)	FAT (g)	SATURATED FAT (g)	CHOLESTEROL (mg)	SODIUM (mg)	FIBER (g)
Frozen dinners *(continued)*										
chicken, fried	1 (11.5 oz.)	601	45	3	27	35	12.0	115	1918	3
chicken, mesquite grilled	1 (10.6 oz.)	380	56	4	23	9	2.5	40	1210	4
chicken & fettuccini Alfredo	1 (16.8 oz.)	619	71	4 ½	19	28	12.5	44	1503	7
chicken Monterey	1 (14.5 oz.)	580	68	4 ½	29	21	7.0	65	1400	4
chicken parmigiana	1 (16 oz.)	660	63	4	30	32	8.0	50	920	5
chicken teriyaki	1 (11.5 oz.)	340	49	3	20	7	2.0	50	1650	3
fish fillet, breaded	1 (10 oz.)	400	51	3	16	15	4.0	45	1300	3
meatloaf	1 (17 oz.)	502	41	2 ½	22	29	11.0	107	1827	5
pork cutlet	1 (10 oz.)	410	37	2 ½	11	24	7.0	34	1034	4
Salisbury steak, w/ gravy & mashed potato	1 (16 oz.)	572	45	3	26	32	16.0	50	1746	7
steak, country fried	1 (16 oz.)	820	63	4	29	50	23.0	70	2260	6
turkey, roasted	1 (11.8 oz.)	519	10	½	71	19	6.5	177	2275	0
veal, w/ vegetables & potato wedges	1 (17.5 oz.)	439	41	2 ½	43	12	3.5	140	1160	8
Frozen dinners, Healthy Choice®										
beef pot roast	1 (11 oz.)	290	45	3	17	5	1.5	40	500	6
country herb chicken	1 (11.4 oz.)	240	34	2	15	5	1.5	30	600	5
lemon pepper fish	1 (10.7 oz.)	310	50	3	14	5	1.0	25	450	5
manicotti formaggio	1 (11.8 oz.)	350	61	4	13	6	3.0	30	570	8
Frozen dinners, Lean Cuisine®										
chicken tuscan	1 (12 oz.)	280	34	2	22	6	2.0	30	780	4
grilled chicken & penne	1 (12 oz.)	330	53	3	18	5	2.0	30	500	6
lemon garlic shrimp	1 (12 oz.)	280	39	2 ½	18	6	3.0	75	830	5
steak tips dijon	1 (12 oz.)	280	35	2	18	7	2.0	30	600	5
Frozen dinners, Smart Ones® Bistro Selections®										
chicken carbonara	1 (9.2 oz.)	260	32	2	21	5	2.0	40	700	2
chicken Santa Fe	1 (9 oz.)	140	11	1	20	3	0.5	30	800	4
Salisbury steak	1 (9 oz.)	200	12	1	20	7	2.5	55	740	4
stuffed turkey breast	1 (9 oz.)	260	39	2 ½	14	5	1.5	20	700	4
Frozen entrées										
chicken à la king	1 (11.5 oz.)	350	45	3	18	11	3.5	45	1150	2
fettuccini Alfredo	1 (11.5 oz.)	424	48	3	13	19	8.5	30	1029	5
manicotti, w/ red sauce	1 (9 oz.)	360	41	3	18	14	6.0	70	920	2
meatloaf, w/ gravy & mashed potato	1 (11.5 oz.)	444	35	2	19	25	10.0	78	1290	4
stuffed peppers, w/ beef	1 (15.5 oz.)	200	21	1 ½	8	9	3.5	25	730	2
Swedish meatballs, w/ pasta	1 (11.5 oz.)	346	40	2 ½	28	9	3.5	62	776	3
Turkey tetrazzini	1 (10 oz.)	439	31	2	21	24	8.0	72	845	2
Hamburger Helper®, box										
beef pasta	1 cup	280	23	1 ½	21	11	4.5	55	760	1

ITEM	AMOUNT	CALORIES	CARBOHYDRATE (g)	CARBOHYDRATE CHOICES	PROTEIN (g)	FAT (g)	SATURATED FAT (g)	CHOLESTEROL (mg)	SODIUM (mg)	FIBER (g)
Hamburger Helper®, box *(continued)*										
cheeseburger macaroni	1 cup	310	27	2	22	12	5.0	60	910	0
chunky taco	1 cup	340	33	2	20	14	5.0	55	880	0
Italian lasagna	1 cup	280	27	2	19	11	4.0	55	900	0
Philly cheesesteak	1 cup	320	28	2	22	13	5.0	55	750	1
tomato basil penne	1 cup	300	31	2	20	11	4.0	55	710	1
Hot Pockets®, frzn.										
cheeseburger	1 (4.5 oz.)	310	38	2 ½	10	12	6.0	25	570	1
chicken melt w/ bacon	1 (4.5 oz.)	300	36	2 ½	11	12	5.0	30	570	2
ham n' cheese	1 (4.5 oz.)	290	36	2 ½	10	12	5.0	30	640	1
meatballs & mozzarella	1 (4.5 oz.)	340	37	2 ½	10	16	7.0	30	570	2
pepperoni pizza	1 (4.5 oz.)	360	33	2	10	21	10.0	15	690	2
Philly steak & cheese	1 (4.5 oz.)	310	37	2 ½	10	13	7.0	30	590	1
Lasagna										
w/ meat	6 oz.	272	28	2	16	11	5.5	40	272	2
w/ vegetables	6 oz.	239	31	2	12	7	4.5	25	284	2
Lean Pockets®, frzn.										
chicken, broccoli & cheddar	1 (4.5 oz.)	250	40	2 ½	10	7	3.0	20	420	3
pepperoni pizza	1 (4.5 oz.)	290	40	2 ½	12	8	4.0	20	610	2
Philly steak & cheese	1 (4.5 oz.)	270	39	2 ½	10	8	4.0	25	540	2
Lo mein, pork	6 oz.	241	18	1	17	12	2.0	36	121	2
Macaroni & cheese										
frzn.	1 (11.5 oz.)	402	55	3 ½	14	13	7.5	19	1275	5
three cheese, box	1 cup	410	48	3	11	3	1.0	10	610	2
Manicotti, w/ red sauce	2 large	580	66	4	20	28	12.0	80	1520	6
Meatballs	1 medium	58	2	0	5	3	1.0	23	83	0
Meatloaf	3 oz.	169	5	0	15	9	3.5	69	101	0
Moussaka	1 cup	238	13	1	17	13	4.5	97	460	4
Pasta Roni®, box										
butter & garlic	1 cup	250	39	2 ½	8	8	2.0	5	690	2
butter & herb Italiano	1 cup	300	41	3	9	11	3.0	5	780	2
cheddar macaroni	1 cup	200	37	2 ½	7	3	1.0	0	510	1
tomato parmesan	1 cup	270	40	2 ½	10	9	3.0	5	840	2
Pepper steak	1 cup	320	6	½	28	20	4.0	70	563	1
Pizza, French bread, frzn.										
cheese	1 (5.2 oz.)	350	42	3	15	14	5.0	15	660	3
pepperoni	1 (5.6 oz.)	420	42	3	18	20	6.0	35	930	3
vegetable	1 (6 oz.)	280	44	3	17	4	1.5	10	480	5
Pizza, frzn.										
cheese	1 (5.2 oz.) slice	341	36	2 ½	15	15	5.5	18	663	2
pepperoni	1 (5.2 oz.) slice	378	35	2	13	20	4.5	18	912	2

COMBINATION FOODS, FROZEN ENTRÉES & MEALS

ITEM	AMOUNT	CALORIES	CARBOHYDRATE (g)	CARBOHYDRATE CHOICES	PROTEIN (g)	FAT (g)	SATURATED FAT (g)	CHOLESTEROL (mg)	SODIUM (mg)	FIBER (g)
Pizza Rolls®, frzn.										
cheese	6 rolls	200	26	2	7	8	2.5	0	480	1
pepperoni	6 rolls	220	24	1 ½	7	11	3.0	10	460	1
Pot pies, frzn.										
beef	1 (7 oz.)	400	38	2 ½	9	23	11.0	30	1000	1
chicken	1 (7 oz.)	381	36	2 ½	11	22	8.5	30	843	3
Ravioli, w/ red sauce										
cheese	6 oz.	232	26	2	10	10	4.5	110	390	2
meat	6 oz.	268	25	1 ½	15	12	4.0	116	122	2
Salmon loaf	3 oz.	168	7	½	14	9	2.5	99	410	0
Salmon patties	1 (4.2 oz.)	259	14	1	16	15	3.5	56	502	1
Sandwiches, w/ bread/bun										
BBQ beef	1 (6.8 oz.)	407	50	3	22	12	5.0	48	828	3
BLT, w/ mayo.	1 (4.7 oz.)	342	32	2	11	19	4.5	22	679	2
bologna & cheese	1 (3.9 oz.)	348	28	2	13	20	8.5	35	936	1
cheeseburger	1 (4.9 oz.)	363	31	2	20	17	6.5	65	632	2
chicken, breaded & fried	1 (7.2 oz.)	492	46	3	34	19	4.0	72	1561	1
chicken, roasted	1 (6.5 oz.)	250	37	2 ½	18	4	1.5	35	781	4
chicken club, w/ mayo.	1 (7.6 oz.)	471	47	3	30	19	4.0	65	922	2
chicken salad, w/ mayo.	1 (4.2 oz.)	396	34	2	11	24	3.0	33	523	2
corned beef & Swiss	1 (5.5 oz.)	427	22	1	28	26	9.5	83	1470	6
egg salad, w/ mayo.	1 (4.4 oz.)	404	33	2	10	26	4.0	164	533	2
grilled cheese	1 (4.5 oz.)	427	32	2	18	25	12.5	57	1238	1
ham & cheese, w/ mustard	1 (5.8 oz.)	396	38	2 ½	23	17	7.5	66	868	2
ham salad, w/ mayo.	1 (4.9 oz.)	383	39	2 ½	11	20	4.5	30	992	1
hamburger	1 (4.9 oz.)	292	29	2	17	12	5.0	45	634	2
hot dog	1 (3.5 oz.)	241	19	1	9	14	5.0	25	732	1
peanut butter & jelly	1 (4 oz.)	390	52	3 ½	12	16	3.0	1	481	3
Reuben, w/ dressing	1 (6.4 oz.)	475	37	2 ½	26	29	6.0	64	1112	2
roast beef, w/ cheese	1 (5.5 oz.)	419	40	2 ½	29	16	8.0	69	1447	1
salami & cheese, w/ mustard	1 (4.1 oz.)	354	27	2	15	21	11.0	40	1066	1
sloppy Joe, beef	1 (6.6 oz.)	392	36	2 ½	24	18	7.0	66	965	3
tuna salad, w/ mayo.	1 (4.6 oz.)	349	38	2 ½	14	15	2.0	14	629	1
turkey	1 (5.8 oz.)	365	31	2	25	15	2.0	45	1675	1
Scalloped potatoes & ham	1 cup	216	26	1 ½	7	9	3.5	15	821	5
Shepherd's pie	1 cup	278	32	2	17	9	2.5	37	312	3
Spaghetti, w/ meatballs	1 cup	362	28	2	18	18	5.0	65	1133	3
SpaghettiO's®, can										
w/ meatballs	1 cup	240	32	2	11	7	2.5	20	600	4
w/ sliced franks	1 cup	220	32	2	9	6	2.5	20	600	4
w/ tomato & cheese sauce	1 cup	170	35	2	6	1	0.5	5	600	3

COMBINATION FOODS, FROZEN ENTRÉES & MEALS

ITEM	AMOUNT	CALORIES	CARBOHYDRATE (g)	CARBOHYDRATE CHOICES	PROTEIN (g)	FAT (g)	SATURATED FAT (g)	CHOLESTEROL (mg)	SODIUM (mg)	FIBER (g)
Stew										
beef, can	1 cup	210	20	1	12	9	4.0	50	1150	3
beef, hmde.	6 oz.	158	14	1	8	8	3.5	22	221	2
chicken, can	1 cup	140	19	1	10	3	1.0	20	910	2
turkey, can	1 cup	140	19	1	10	3	1.0	20	910	2
Stuffed cabbage rolls	1 (8.1 oz.)	186	17	1	12	8	3.0	37	520	2
Stuffed green peppers	1 (6.1 oz.)	229	18	1	12	12	5.5	37	233	1
Stuffed shells, w/ red sauce	2 (3 oz.)	357	35	2	23	14	7.0	0	850	4
Suddenly Salad®										
classic	¾ cup	250	38	2 ½	6	8	1.0	0	820	1
creamy Italian	¾ cup	350	36	2 ½	7	20	2.5	15	540	2
ranch & bacon	¾ cup	350	34	2	6	21	2.0	15	470	2
Sweet & sour pork	1 cup	231	25	1 ½	15	8	2.0	39	839	2
Tacos, soft shell										
beef	1 (4 oz.)	248	22	1 ½	13	12	5.0	32	717	3
chicken	1 (4 oz.)	190	19	1	14	6	3.0	30	760	4
Tamales	1 (2.4 oz.)	104	12	1	4	4	1.5	12	291	2
Tortellini, w/ red sauce										
cheese	1 cup	394	59	4	17	10	4.0	45	665	4
meat	1 cup	312	47	3	13	8	4.0	40	784	4
Tuna Helper®, box										
creamy broccoli	1 cup	260	29	2	15	10	3.0	25	830	1
creamy parmesan	1 cup	270	30	2	15	10	3.0	25	810	1
Veal Marsala	6 oz.	473	11	1	21	35	15.0	124	254	0
Veal parmigiana	6 oz.	350	21	1 ½	27	17	6.0	86	1672	2
Veal scallopini	6 oz.	421	3	0	32	30	8.5	114	493	1
Welsh rarebit, frzn.	1 (2.2 oz.)	120	5	0	5	9	4.0	20	280	0
Yorkshire pudding	2 oz.	118	14	1	4	6	2.5	43	335	1
Ziti, w/ meat sauce	6 oz.	272	28	2	16	11	5.5	40	272	2

CONDIMENTS, SAUCES & BAKING INGREDIENTS
Condiments & Sauces

ITEM	AMOUNT	CALORIES	CARBOHYDRATE (g)	CARBOHYDRATE CHOICES	PROTEIN (g)	FAT (g)	SATURATED FAT (g)	CHOLESTEROL (mg)	SODIUM (mg)	FIBER (g)
Alfredo sauce	¼ cup	180	3	0	3	18	7.0	25	600	0
BBQ sauce	1 T.	20	4	0	0	0	0.0	0	212	0
Béarnaise sauce	2 T.	80	0	0	1	8	5.0	58	112	0
Béchamel sauce	2 T.	35	2	0	0	3	2.0	8	287	0
Catsup/ketchup	1 T.	15	4	0	0	0	0.0	0	167	0
Cheese sauce	2 T.	52	3	0	1	4	1.0	1	316	0
Chili sauce	2 T.	30	8	½	0	0	0.0	0	360	0
Chipotle grilling sauce	2 T.	60	14	1	0	0	0.0	0	510	0
Chipotle hot sauce	1 tsp.	0	0	0	0	0	0.0	0	85	0
Chutney	2 T.	50	11	1	0	1	0.0	0	15	1

CONDIMENTS, SAUCES & BAKING INGREDIENTS

Condiments & Sauces

ITEM	AMOUNT	CALORIES	CARBOHYDRATE (g)	CARBOHYDRATE CHOICES	PROTEIN (g)	FAT (g)	SATURATED FAT (g)	CHOLESTEROL (mg)	SODIUM (mg)	FIBER (g)
Clam sauce										
red	½ cup	60	8	½	4	1	0.0	10	350	1
white	½ cup	140	5	0	7	10	1.5	15	510	0
Cocktail sauce	2 T.	30	7	½	1	0	0.0	0	400	1
Cranberry-orange relish	2 T.	61	16	1	0	0	0.0	0	11	0
Cranberry sauce	2 T.	52	13	1	0	0	0.0	0	10	0
Duck sauce	2 T.	47	12	1	0	0	0.0	0	98	0
Enchilada sauce										
green	2 T.	13	2	0	0	1	0.0	0	170	0
red	2 T.	13	3	0	1	0	0.0	0	275	1
Fish sauce	1 T.	6	1	0	1	0	0.0	0	1390	0
Hoisin sauce	1 T.	35	7	½	1	1	0.0	0	258	0
Hollandaise sauce	2 T.	85	0	0	1	9	5.0	90	78	0
Horseradish	1 T.	7	2	0	0	0	0.0	0	47	0
Horseradish sauce	1 T.	60	3	0	0	5	0.0	15	105	0
Jerk sauce	2 T.	70	18	1	0	0	0.0	0	200	0
Lobster sauce	1 T.	24	1	0	1	2	0.5	11	43	0
Manwich® sauce	¼ cup	40	9	½	0	0	0.0	0	410	2
Mole poblano sauce	2 T.	50	4	0	1	3	1.0	0	41	1
Mornay sauce	2 T.	90	3	0	3	8	3.5	40	196	0
Mustard										
brown/yellow	1 tsp.	0	0	0	0	0	0.0	0	55	0
Dijon	1 tsp.	5	0	0	0	0	0.0	0	120	0
honey	1 tsp.	10	1	0	0	0	0.0	0	20	0
Olives										
black	5	25	1	0	0	2	0.5	0	192	1
green, w/ pimento	5	21	0	0	0	2	0.5	0	413	0
Oyster sauce	1 T.	30	6	½	0	0	0.0	0	900	0
Pasta sauce, red										
arrabbiata, Bertoli®	½ cup	60	11	1	1	2	0.0	0	450	2
four cheese, Classico®	½ cup	80	12	1	2	3	1.0	0	460	3
fradiavolo	½ cup	70	4	0	5	4	1.0	0	380	2
garden combination, Ragu®	½ cup	90	14	1	2	3	0.0	0	460	2
light, Ragú®	½ cup	50	11	1	2	0	0.0	0	360	2
marinara, hmde.	½ cup	93	14	1	2	3	0.5	0	601	1
marinara, Newman's Own®	½ cup	70	12	1	2	2	0.0	0	510	3
meat flavored, Ragú®	½ cup	70	9	½	2	3	0.5	0	470	2
primavera	½ cup	70	11	1	5	3	0.0	0	500	2
sausage, Bertolli®	½ cup	100	15	1	3	3	0.5	0	580	3
Sockarooni®, Newman's Own®	½ cup	70	12	1	2	2	0.0	0	520	0
tomato & basil, Barilla®	½ cup	80	13	1	2	2	0.0	0	520	3
traditional, Prego®	½ cup	70	13	1	2	2	0.0	0	480	3

CONDIMENTS, SAUCES & BAKING INGREDIENTS

Condiments & Sauces

ITEM	AMOUNT	CALORIES	CARBOHYDRATE (g)	CARBOHYDRATE CHOICES	PROTEIN (g)	FAT (g)	SATURATED FAT (g)	CHOLESTEROL (mg)	SODIUM (mg)	FIBER (g)
Pasta sauce, red *(continued)*										
traditional, Ragú®	½ cup	70	10	½	2	3	0.0	0	480	2
vodka, Classico®	½ cup	100	11	1	3	5	2.0	10	420	3
w/ meat, hmde.	½ cup	144	11	1	8	8	2.5	23	434	2
Peanut sauce	2 T.	94	4	0	4	8	1.5	0	73	1
Pesto sauce	2 T.	155	2	0	6	14	4.0	10	238	1
Pickles										
bread & butter	3 chips	18	5	0	0	0	0.0	0	103	0
dill	1 medium	4	1	0	0	0	0.0	0	226	0
sweet	1 medium	28	7	½	0	0	0.0	0	160	0
Pico de gallo	2 T.	12	2	0	0	0	0.0	0	191	0
Pizza sauce	¼ cup	30	6	½	1	0	0.0	0	340	1
Plum sauce	2 T.	70	16	1	0	0	0.0	0	205	0
Relish, sweet pickle	1 T.	20	5	0	0	0	0.0	0	124	0
Salsa	2 T.	15	2	0	0	0	0.0	0	240	1
Salt	1 tsp.	0	0	0	0	0	0.0	0	2325	0
Sauerkraut, can	2 T.	6	1	0	0	0	0.0	0	195	1
Soy sauce										
lite	1 T.	15	2	0	1	0	0.0	0	505	0
regular	1 T.	11	2	0	1	0	0.0	0	1315	0
Spices, salt free	¼ tsp.	0	0	0	0	0	0.0	0	0	0
Steak sauce										
A.1.®	1 T.	15	3	0	0	0	0.0	0	280	0
Heinz 57®	1 T.	20	4	0	0	0	0.0	0	190	0
Stir-fry sauce	1 T.	15	3	0	1	0	0.0	0	530	0
Sweet & sour sauce	1 T.	18	5	0	0	0	0.0	0	95	0
Szechuan sauce	1 T.	20	4	0	0	1	0.0	0	520	0
Tabasco® sauce	1 tsp.	0	0	0	0	0	0.0	0	35	0
Taco sauce	1 T.	10	1	0	0	0	0.0	0	60	0
Tamari sauce	1 T.	11	1	0	2	0	0.0	0	1005	0
Tartar sauce	1 T.	40	2	0	0	4	0.5	5	150	0
Teriyaki sauce	1 T.	15	3	0	1	0	0.0	0	690	0
Tomato sauce, can	½ cup	29	7	½	2	0	0.0	0	642	2
Vinegar										
balsamic	1 T.	10	2	0	0	0	0.0	0	4	0
cider/white	1 T.	3	0	0	0	0	0.0	0	1	0
raspberry/red wine	1 T.	0	0	0	0	0	0.0	0	2	0
White cream sauce	2 T.	30	2	0	1	2	1.0	3	140	0
Worcestershire sauce	1 tsp.	4	1	0	0	0	0.0	0	56	0

CONDIMENTS, SAUCES & BAKING INGREDIENTS

Baking Ingredients

ITEM	AMOUNT	CALORIES	CARBOHYDRATE (g)	CARBOHYDRATE CHOICES	PROTEIN (g)	FAT (g)	SATURATED FAT (g)	CHOLESTEROL (mg)	SODIUM (mg)	FIBER (g)
Baking Ingredients										
Agave nectar										
amber	1 T.	60	16	1	0	0	0.0	0	0	1
light	1 T.	60	16	1	0	0	0.0	0	0	0
Baking powder	¼ tsp.	0	0	0	0	0	0.0	0	100	0
Baking soda	¼ tsp.	0	0	0	0	0	0.0	0	315	0
Bisquick®, dry										
gluten free	⅓ cup	140	31	2	2	1	0.0	0	340	0
reduced fat	⅓ cup	140	27	2	3	3	0.0	0	340	0
regular	⅓ cup	160	26	2	3	5	1.0	0	410	1
Bread crumbs										
plain	¼ cup	110	20	1	4	2	0.5	0	220	1
seasoned	¼ cup	110	20	1	4	2	0.5	0	470	1
Butterscotch chips	1 T.	80	9	½	0	4	3.5	0	15	0
Carob chips, unsweetened	1 T.	70	8	½	2	3	3.0	0	65	0
Chocolate, baking										
semi-sweet	1 oz.	140	16	1	1	9	5.0	0	0	2
unsweetened	1 oz.	140	8	½	4	14	9.0	0	0	4
Chocolate chips										
milk chocolate	1 T.	70	9	½	0	4	2.5	0	5	0
semi-sweet	1 T.	70	9	½	0	4	2.5	0	0	0
Cocoa powder	1 T.	15	3	0	1	1	0.0	0	0	1
Corn flake crumbs	¼ cup	80	19	1	1	0	0.0	0	160	0
Corn starch	1 T.	30	7	½	0	0	0.0	0	1	0
Corn syrup, dark/light	1 T.	59	16	1	0	0	0.0	0	32	0
Cornmeal	2 T.	55	12	1	1	1	0.0	0	5	1
Flour										
all purpose/white	1 cup	455	95	6	13	1	0.0	0	3	3
bread	1 cup	495	99	6 ½	16	2	0.5	0	3	3
buckwheat	1 cup	348	61	3 ½	15	3	0.0	0	0	18
cake	1 cup	496	107	7	11	1	0.0	0	3	2
carob	1 cup	229	92	5	5	1	0.0	0	36	41
corn	1 cup	416	87	5	11	4	0.5	0	6	15
potato	1 cup	571	133	8 ½	11	1	0.0	0	88	9
rice, white	1 cup	578	127	8 ½	9	2	0.5	0	0	4
rye, medium	1 cup	361	79	5	10	2	0.0	0	3	15
soy	1 cup	369	27	1 ½	32	18	2.5	0	11	8
soy, fat free	1 cup	330	38	2	47	1	0.0	0	20	18
white, self-rising	1 cup	443	93	6	12	1	0.0	0	1588	3
whole wheat	1 cup	407	87	5	16	2	0.5	0	6	15
Graham cracker crumbs	3 T.	70	13	1	1	2	0.0	0	140	1
Honey	1 T.	64	17	1	0	0	0.0	0	1	0

CONDIMENTS, SAUCES & BAKING INGREDIENTS

Baking Ingredients

ITEM	AMOUNT	CALORIES	CARBOHYDRATE (g)	CARBOHYDRATE CHOICES	PROTEIN (g)	FAT (g)	SATURATED FAT (g)	CHOLESTEROL (mg)	SODIUM (mg)	FIBER (g)
Lighter Bake™	1 T.	35	9	½	0	0	0.0	0	0	0
Matzo meal, unsalted	2 T.	65	14	1	2	0	0.0	0	0	0
Molasses	1 T.	58	15	1	0	0	0.0	0	7	0
Phyllo dough	3 sheets	170	30	2	4	3	1.0	0	275	1
Pie crusts										
graham	1/8 pie	110	14	1	1	5	1.0	0	115	1
graham, chocolate	1/8 pie	100	14	1	1	5	1.0	0	110	0
graham, reduced fat	1/8 pie	90	15	1	1	4	0.5	0	100	0
pastry, double, hmde.	1/8 pie	227	21	1 ½	3	15	3.5	0	234	2
pastry, single, hmde.	1/8 pie	119	11	1	1	8	2.0	0	122	0
Pie fillings										
apple	1/3 cup	86	22	1 ½	0	0	0.0	0	37	1
blueberry	1/3 cup	90	23	1 ½	0	0	0.0	0	50	1
cherry	1/3 cup	101	25	1 ½	0	0	0.0	0	16	1
lemon	1/3 cup	130	28	2	0	2	0.0	0	120	0
pumpkin	1/3 cup	90	20	1	1	1	0.0	0	120	3
Shake 'n Bake®, box	1/8 pkt.	40	7	½	0	1	0.0	0	220	0
Sugar										
brown/raw/white	1 cup	774	200	13	0	0	0.0	0	2	0
powdered	1 cup	467	119	8	0	0	0.0	0	1	0
Yeast	1 pkt.	0	0	0	0	0	0.0	0	0	0

CRACKERS, DIPS & SNACK FOODS

Crackers

ITEM	AMOUNT	CALORIES	CARBOHYDRATE (g)	CARBOHYDRATE CHOICES	PROTEIN (g)	FAT (g)	SATURATED FAT (g)	CHOLESTEROL (mg)	SODIUM (mg)	FIBER (g)
Ak-mak®	5	110	20	1	5	2	0.0	0	140	4
All-Bran®	18	130	19	1	2	6	1.0	0	230	5
Animal	10	130	22	1 ½	2	4	1.0	0	140	0
Better Cheddars®	22	160	18	1	3	8	1.5	5	360	1
Cheese, w/ peanut butter	6	190	23	1 ½	4	10	1.5	0	330	1
Cheese Nips®	29	150	19	1	3	6	1.5	0	340	0
Cheez-It®										
original, reduced fat	29	130	20	1	4	5	1.0	0	250	0
original, regular	27	150	17	1	3	8	2.0	0	230	0
regular, white cheddar	25	150	19	1	3	8	2.0	0	210	0
Chicken In A Biskit®	12	160	19	1	2	8	1.5	0	310	1
Club®										
multi-grain	4	70	9	½	1	3	0.0	0	120	0
original, minis	17	70	10	½	0	3	0.5	0	150	0
original, regular	4	70	9	½	0	3	0.5	0	125	0
reduced fat	5	70	12	1	1	2	0.0	0	150	0
Gold Fish®										
cheddar	55	140	20	1	4	5	1.0	0	250	0

CRACKERS, DIPS & SNACK FOODS
Crackers

ITEM	AMOUNT	CALORIES	CARBOHYDRATE (g)	CARBOHYDRATE CHOICES	PROTEIN (g)	FAT (g)	SATURATED FAT (g)	CHOLESTEROL (mg)	SODIUM (mg)	FIBER (g)
Gold Fish® *(continued)*										
chocolate grahams	50	130	22	1 ½	2	4	1.0	0	125	2
original, saltine	55	150	20	1	3	6	0.5	0	230	0
parmesan	60	130	20	1	4	4	1.0	0	280	0
pizza	55	140	20	1	3	5	1.0	0	230	0
pretzel	43	130	24	1 ½	3	3	0.5	0	430	0
Graham										
reduced fat	2 sheets	130	24	1 ½	2	3	0.5	0	190	1
regular	2 sheets	130	24	1 ½	2	3	0.5	0	190	1
Matzos, lightly salted	1 sheet	110	23	1 ½	3	1	0.0	0	100	1
Melba snacks	5	60	12	1	2	1	0.0	0	135	2
Milk crackers	1	50	8	½	1	2	0.5	1	65	0
Oyster	22	60	11	1	1	2	0.0	0	170	0
Popchips™	23	120	20	1	1	4	0.0	0	280	1
Rice	19	120	26	2	2	0	0.0	0	90	1
Ritz®										
original, low sodium	5	80	10	½	1	4	1.0	0	35	0
original, reduced fat	5	70	11	1	1	2	0.0	0	150	0
original, regular	5	80	10	½	1	5	1.0	0	125	0
whole wheat, regular	5	70	11	1	1	3	0.5	0	120	0
Ritz® cracker sandwiches										
w/ cheese	6	200	21	1 ½	2	12	3.0	0	440	0
w/ peanut butter	6	200	21	1 ½	4	11	1.5	0	400	1
Ritz Bits® sandwiches										
w/ cheese	13	150	17	1	2	9	3.0	0	250	0
w/ peanut butter	12	140	16	1	3	8	1.5	0	230	1
Saltines										
fat free	5	60	12	1	1	0	0.0	0	170	0
reduced sodium	5	70	11	1	1	2	0.0	0	95	0
regular	5	60	11	1	1	2	0.0	0	190	0
Seasoned Ry Krisp®	2	60	10	½	1	2	0.0	0	90	3
Sociables®	5	70	9	½	1	4	0.5	0	140	0
Special K Crackers™										
multi-grain	24	120	23	1 ½	3	3	0.0	0	250	3
savory herb	24	120	22	1 ½	3	3	0.0	0	240	3
Table Water®	5	70	13	1	2	2	0.5	0	100	0
Teddy Grahams®										
chocolate	24	130	22	1 ½	2	5	1.0	0	160	2
cinnamon	24	130	23	1 ½	2	4	1.0	0	150	1
honey	24	130	23	1 ½	2	4	1.0	0	150	1

CRACKERS, DIPS & SNACK FOODS

Snack Foods

ITEM	AMOUNT	CALORIES	CARBOHYDRATE (g)	CARBOHYDRATE CHOICES	PROTEIN (g)	FAT (g)	SATURATED FAT (g)	CHOLESTEROL (mg)	SODIUM (mg)	FIBER (g)
Toasteds®										
buttercrisp	5	80	10	½	0	4	0.5	0	150	0
wheat	5	70	11	1	1	3	0.5	0	140	0
Town House®										
flipsides pretzel crackers	5	70	10	½	1	4	0.5	0	190	0
multi-grain toppers	3	70	10	½	1	3	0.0	0	120	0
original	5	80	10	½	0	5	1.0	0	130	0
reduced fat	6	60	11	1	1	2	0.0	0	160	0
wheat	5	80	10	½	1	4	0.5	0	170	0
Triscuit®										
original	6	120	20	1	3	5	0.5	0	180	3
reduced fat	7	120	23	1 ½	3	3	0.0	0	160	3
Vegetable Thins®	21	150	19	1	2	7	2.0	0	320	1
Wasa®										
Crisp'n Light®	3	60	13	1	2	0	0.0	0	95	2
rye	1	30	7	½	0	0	0.0	0	35	2
sourdough	1	35	9	½	1	0	0.0	0	45	2
whole grain	1	40	10	½	1	0	0.0	0	50	2
Wheat Thins®										
low sodium	16	150	23	1 ½	2	5	1.0	0	60	2
multigrain	15	140	22	1 ½	3	5	0.5	0	200	3
original, regular	16	140	22	1 ½	2	5	1.0	0	230	2
ranch	15	140	21	1 ½	2	5	1.0	0	190	2
reduced fat	16	130	22	1 ½	2	4	0.5	0	230	2
Wheatables®										
original golden wheat	17	140	20	1	2	6	1.5	0	210	1
toasted honey wheat	17	140	20	1	2	6	1.5	0	200	1
Dips										
Bean	2 T.	40	5	0	2	1	0.0	0	170	1
Caramel apple	2 T.	150	24	1 ½	1	5	4.0	5	75	1
Cheese	2 T.	50	3	0	1	4	1.0	0	250	0
Cream cheese fruit dip	2 T.	70	10	½	0	3	2.0	15	85	0
French onion	2 T.	50	2	0	1	5	2.0	0	230	0
Garlic & herb	2 T.	100	2	0	2	9	6.0	25	75	0
Marshmallow éclair	2 T.	97	11	1	1	5	3.5	17	56	0
Ranch	2 T.	60	1	0	1	5	2.5	0	240	0
Salsa, w/ cheese	2 T.	40	5	0	0	3	1.0	0	280	0
Spinach	2 T.	140	3	0	0	14	2.0	10	200	0
Snack Foods										
Bagel chips	7 medium	140	17	1	3	6	3.0	0	70	1

CRACKERS, DIPS & SNACK FOODS
Snack Foods

ITEM	AMOUNT	CALORIES	CARBOHYDRATE (g)	CARBOHYDRATE CHOICES	PROTEIN (g)	FAT (g)	SATURATED FAT (g)	CHOLESTEROL (mg)	SODIUM (mg)	FIBER (g)
Snack Foods *(continued)*										
Bugles®, original	1⅓ cups	160	18	1	1	9	8.0	0	310	0
Cheerios® snack mix	⅔ cup	120	21	1 ½	2	3	0.5	0	240	2
Cheetos®										
crunchy	21	160	15	1	2	10	2.0	0	290	0
puffs	13	160	13	1	2	10	2.0	0	350	0
Cheez Doodles®										
crunchy	½ cup	150	17	1	1	9	2.5	0	220	0
puffed	23	150	17	1	2	8	2.0	0	320	0
Cheez-It® party mix	½ cup	130	20	1	3	5	1.0	0	330	1
Chex Mix®, traditional	½ cup	120	20	1	2	4	1.0	0	210	1
Combos®										
cheddar, w/ cracker	⅓ cup	140	18	1	2	6	3.0	0	290	0
cheddar, w/ pretzel	⅓ cup	130	19	1	3	5	3.0	0	440	0
Cornnuts®										
barbecue	⅓ cup	130	20	1	2	5	0.5	0	170	2
original	⅓ cup	120	20	1	3	5	0.5	0	180	2
Cracker Jack®	½ cup	120	23	1 ½	2	2	0.0	0	70	1
Doritos® nacho chips										
cool ranch	12	150	18	1	2	8	1.0	0	180	2
nacho cheese	11	150	17	1	2	8	1.5	0	180	1
spicy sweet chili	11	140	18	1	2	7	1.0	0	270	1
Fritos® corn chips	32	160	16	1	2	10	1.5	0	160	1
Funyuns®	13	140	18	1	2	7	1.0	0	240	0
Jax®	23	140	17	1	2	7	1.0	0	300	0
Popcorn										
air popped	3 cups	93	19	1	3	1	0.0	0	2	3
caramel, fat free	1 cup	112	27	2	1	0	0.0	0	150	2
caramel, regular	1 cup	130	24	1 ½	1	4	1.5	0	50	1
caramel & peanuts	1 cup	170	34	2	3	3	0.5	0	125	2
cheddar cheese	3 cups	174	17	1	3	11	2.0	4	293	3
Jiffy Pop®	3 cups	105	14	1	2	5	1.0	0	165	2
oil popped, salted	3 cups	165	19	1	3	9	1.5	0	292	3
Smartfood®, white cheddar	1¾ cups	160	14	1	3	10	2.0	0	290	2
toffee, fat free	¾ cup	110	26	2	1	0	0.0	0	85	1
Popcorn, microwave										
butter	3 cups	105	12	1	2	8	1.5	0	180	3
kettle corn	3 cups	90	10	½	1	6	3.0	0	60	2
light	3 cups	60	12	1	2	3	0.5	0	145	2
SmartPop!®	3 cups	50	12	1	2	1	0.0	0	110	2
Popcorn cakes										
caramel	1 (4 inch)	50	11	1	1	0	0.0	0	30	0

ITEM	AMOUNT	CALORIES	CARBOHYDRATE (g)	CARBOHYDRATE CHOICES	PROTEIN (g)	FAT (g)	SATURATED FAT (g)	CHOLESTEROL (mg)	SODIUM (mg)	FIBER (g)
Popcorn cakes *(continued)*										
plain	1 (4 inch)	40	8	½	1	0	0.0	0	40	0
white cheddar	1 (4 inch)	45	8	½	1	0	0.0	0	65	0
Pork rinds	9	80	0	0	7	5	2.5	20	310	0
Potato chips										
baked	15	110	23	1 ½	2	2	0.0	0	180	2
BBQ	15	150	15	1	2	10	1.0	0	200	1
regular	15	150	15	1	2	10	1.0	0	180	1
Potato sticks	1 cup	250	23	1 ½	3	16	6.5	0	270	1
Pretzels										
chocolate covered	8 small	130	20	1	2	5	3.0	0	135	1
rods	2	110	23	1 ½	3	0	0.0	0	240	1
sourdough, hard	1 large	100	21	1 ½	2	1	0.0	0	500	1
thin twists	20 small	110	25	1 ½	3	0	0.0	0	250	0
thin twists	11 large	110	23	1 ½	3	0	0.0	0	330	0
yogurt covered	8 small	130	21	1 ½	1	5	4.0	0	170	0
Pringles® potato crisps										
BBQ, regular	16	150	15	1	1	9	2.5	0	140	1
multi grain	16	150	16	1	1	8	2.0	0	150	1
original, light	15	70	15	1	1	0	0.0	0	160	1
original, regular	16	150	15	1	1	9	2.5	0	150	1
sour cream & onion	16	150	15	1	1	9	2.5	0	170	1
Rice cakes										
mini, caramel	6 (2 inch)	60	13	1	1	0	0.0	0	30	1
mini, soy	6 (2 inch)	70	9	½	5	2	0.0	0	200	2
regular, chocolate	1 (4 inch)	60	11	1	1	1	0.0	0	30	0
regular, plain	1 (4 inch)	35	7	½	2	0	0.0	0	15	0
Sesame sticks	12 small	130	19	1	3	5	1.0	0	290	2
Sun Chips®, original	16	140	19	1	2	6	1.0	0	120	3
Tostitos® tortilla chips										
bite size, regular	24	140	18	1	2	7	1.0	0	110	2
blue/yellow corn	6	140	19	1	2	6	0.5	0	80	1
crispy rounds	13	140	18	1	2	7	1.0	0	120	2
dipping strips	11	150	19	1	2	7	1.0	0	115	2
hint of lime	6	150	18	1	2	7	1.0	0	125	2
restaurant style, regular	7	140	19	1	2	7	1.0	0	115	2
Scoops!®	12	140	19	1	2	7	1.0	0	120	2
Veggie Stix®, original	1 oz.	130	20	1	1	5	1.0	0	310	0
Wheat Nuts®										
low sodium	⅓ cup	200	5	0	4	19	3.0	0	30	1
original	⅓ cup	200	5	0	4	19	3.0	0	190	1

DESSERTS, SWEETS & TOPPINGS
Bars

ITEM	AMOUNT	CALORIES	CARBOHYDRATE (g)	CARBOHYDRATE CHOICES	PROTEIN (g)	FAT (g)	SATURATED FAT (g)	CHOLESTEROL (mg)	SODIUM (mg)	FIBER (g)
DESSERTS, SWEETS & TOPPINGS										
Bars										
Brownies, chocolate										
fat free, mix	1 (2 inch)	181	42	3	2	0	0.0	0	272	1
regular, w/ nuts	1 (2 inch)	180	21	1 ½	2	10	1.5	19	96	0
regular, w/o nuts	1 (2 inch)	170	25	1 ½	2	8	1.0	19	106	0
turtle, regular	1 (2 inch)	170	23	1 ½	1	8	1.5	12	124	0
Kudos®, peanut butter	1 (1 oz.)	130	18	1	2	6	3.0	0	75	1
Lemon	1 (2 inch)	160	29	2	1	4	1.0	35	92	1
Nutty Bars®	1 (1 oz.)	155	17	1	2	9	3.5	0	58	1
Rice Krispies Treats®										
chocolatey drizzle	1 (0.8 oz.)	100	17	1	0	3	1.0	0	95	0
original	1 (0.8 oz.)	90	17	1	0	3	1.0	0	105	0
Seven layer	1 (2 inch)	224	24	1 ½	4	14	7.0	18	114	1
Cakes, Pastries & Sweet Breads										
Angel food cake	1/12 cake	140	32	2	4	0	0.0	0	370	0
Apple dumplings	1 (3 oz.)	233	30	2	2	12	2.5	0	256	2
Apple fritters	1 (1 oz.)	90	12	1	2	4	1.0	0	96	1
Baklava	1 (2 inch)	336	29	2	5	23	9.5	36	293	2
Banana bread	1 (2 oz.)	185	31	2	2	6	1.5	24	171	1
Black forest cake	1/12 cake	298	35	2	3	16	3.0	49	238	6
Caramel rolls	1 (1.7 oz.)	170	24	1 ½	2	7	1.5	0	330	1
Carrot cake, iced	1 (4 oz.)	447	58	4	3	24	5.5	56	367	2
Cheesecake										
amaretto	1 (3 oz.)	290	20	1	6	21	11.0	105	170	0
chocolate	1 (3 oz.)	322	29	2	5	22	11.0	75	183	0
plain, New York style	1 (3 oz.)	273	22	1 ½	5	19	8.5	47	176	0
Chocolate cake, iced	1/12 cake	262	41	3	3	11	2.5	21	193	1
Cinnamon rolls	1 (3 oz.)	339	45	3	6	15	4.0	49	322	2
Cobblers, fruit	1 (3 inch)	174	21	1 ½	1	9	4.0	0	80	1
Coffeecake										
cinnamon, w/ icing	1 (2 oz.)	267	27	2	3	16	3.0	32	171	1
plain, w/ crumb topping	1 (2 oz.)	237	27	2	4	13	3.5	18	199	1
Cream puffs	1 (4 oz.)	293	26	2	8	18	4.0	152	387	1
Crepes, fruit filled	1 (4 oz.)	211	30	2	5	8	2.0	88	104	2
Crisps, fruit	1 (3 inch)	163	27	2	2	6	3.0	11	89	2
Cupcakes, iced										
chocolate, light	1 (1.5 oz.)	131	29	2	2	2	0.5	0	178	2
chocolate, regular	1 (1.5 oz.)	156	28	2	2	4	1.0	7	191	1
chocolate filled, regular	1 (1.8 oz.)	180	31	2	1	6	3.0	5	290	1
vanilla filled, regular	1 (1.9 oz.)	200	34	2	2	7	3.0	10	180	1

DESSERTS, SWEETS & TOPPINGS
Cakes, Pastries & Sweet Breads

ITEM	AMOUNT	CALORIES	CARBOHYDRATE (g)	CARBOHYDRATE CHOICES	PROTEIN (g)	FAT (g)	SATURATED FAT (g)	CHOLESTEROL (mg)	SODIUM (mg)	FIBER (g)
Danish										
cheese	1 (2.5 oz.)	265	26	2	6	16	5.0	11	319	1
fruit	1 (2.5 oz.)	252	34	2	4	12	2.5	14	251	1
Devil Dogs®	1 (1.6 oz.)	160	29	2	2	4	2.0	0	150	1
Ding Dongs®	1 (1.4 oz.)	180	24	1 ½	2	10	6.5	5	115	1
Doughnuts										
cake, plain	1 medium	300	28	2	4	19	5.0	25	330	1
holes, glazed	5 medium	200	27	2	3	9	2.0	0	220	1
raised, glazed	1 medium	180	25	1 ½	3	8	1.5	0	250	1
Eclairs, chocolate	1 (5 inch)	262	24	1 ½	6	16	4.0	127	337	1
Funnel cake	1 (6 inch)	278	29	2	7	14	2.5	63	117	1
Funny Bones®	1 (1.3 oz.)	155	19	1	3	8	5.0	0	130	1
Gingerbread cake	1 (3 inch)	263	36	2 ½	3	12	3.0	24	242	1
Ho Hos®	1 (1 oz.)	120	18	1	1	6	4.0	10	75	0
Honey buns, iced	1 (1.8 oz.)	220	26	2	3	12	6.0	0	170	1
Lemon cake, iced	1 (4 oz.)	374	55	3 ½	3	16	4.5	45	322	0
Marble cake, iced	1/12 cake	377	61	4	4	14	5.5	47	300	1
Marshmallow pies	1 (1.5 oz.)	179	29	2	2	7	2.0	0	71	1
Pecan spin rolls	1 (1 oz.)	100	16	1	1	4	1.5	0	65	0
Pineapple upside down cake	1 (3 inch)	367	58	4	4	14	3.5	25	366	1
Pop Tart®										
frosted	1 (1.8 oz.)	200	38	2 ½	2	5	1.5	0	170	0
unfrosted	1 (1.8 oz.)	210	37	2 ½	2	5	2.0	0	180	0
Pound cake	1/12 cake	110	13	1	1	6	3.0	40	90	0
Pumpkin bread	1 (2 oz.)	176	27	2	2	7	0.5	24	220	1
Ring Dings®	1 (1.4 oz.)	165	22	1 ½	1	9	6.0	0	115	1
Snow balls	1 (2.1 oz.)	220	35	2	2	8	4.5	15	190	1
Spice cake, iced	1 (4 oz.)	383	65	4	5	12	3.5	52	292	1
Sponge cake	1/12 cake	187	36	2 ½	5	3	1.0	107	144	0
Strudel, w/ fruit	1 (2.5 oz.)	178	33	2	3	5	1.0	13	91	2
SuzyQ's®	1 (2 oz.)	220	34	2	2	9	4.5	10	270	1
Toaster Strudel™	1 (1.9 oz.)	180	27	2	3	7	3.0	5	190	0
Turnovers, w/ fruit	1 (3 oz.)	297	45	3	4	12	3.0	0	289	2
Twinkies®	1 (1.5 oz.)	150	27	2	1	5	2.5	20	220	0
Yankee Doodles®	1 (1.0 oz.)	100	16	1	1	4	1.5	0	110	0
Yellow cake, iced	1/12 cake	239	38	2 ½	2	9	1.5	35	220	0
Yodels®	1 (1.1 oz.)	135	19	1	1	7	4.5	5	70	1
Zingers®	1 (1.4 oz.)	150	25	1 ½	1	5	2.5	10	140	0
Cookies										
Arrowroot biscuit	1	30	5	0	0	1	0.0	0	45	0

DESSERTS, SWEETS & TOPPINGS
Cookies

ITEM	AMOUNT	CALORIES	CARBOHYDRATE (g)	CARBOHYDRATE CHOICES	PROTEIN (g)	FAT (g)	SATURATED FAT (g)	CHOLESTEROL (mg)	SODIUM (mg)	FIBER (g)
Biscotti										
almond	1 medium	90	14	1	2	3	1.0	20	65	0
chocolate almond	1 medium	110	17	1	2	5	2.0	20	65	1
chocolate dipped	1 medium	110	17	1	2	5	2.0	20	70	1
toffee almond dipped	1 medium	110	17	1	2	5	2.0	20	75	0
Chocolate chip										
Chips Ahoy!®, chewy	1	60	9	½	1	3	1.5	0	43	0
Chips Ahoy!®, chunky	1	80	10	½	1	4	1.5	0	55	0
Chips Ahoy!®, reduced fat	1	47	8	½	1	2	1.0	0	50	0
Chips Ahoy!®, regular	1	53	7	½	1	3	1.0	0	37	0
hmde.	1 (2 inch)	78	9	½	1	5	2.5	11	55	0
Chocolate wafers	1	28	5	0	0	1	0.5	0	44	0
E. L. Fudge®, original	1	90	13	1	0	4	1.0	0	50	0
Fig Newtons®										
fat free	1	45	11	1	1	0	0.0	0	63	1
regular	1	55	11	1	1	1	0.0	0	60	1
Fudge stripes	1	53	7	½	1	2	2.0	0	37	0
Ginger snaps	1	30	6	½	0	1	0.5	0	48	0
Girl Scout Cookies®										
Caramel deLites®	1	70	10	½	1	4	3.0	0	43	1
Lemonades™	1	75	11	1	1	4	2.0	0	40	0
Peanut Butter Patties®	1	65	7	½	1	4	2.5	0	55	0
Peanut Butter Sandwich	1	53	9	½	1	2	1.0	0	45	0
Shortbread	1	30	5	0	0	1	0.5	0	26	0
Thanks-A-Lot™	1	75	11	1	1	3	2.0	0	55	0
Thin Mints	1	40	0	½	0	2	1.5	0	34	0
Iced animal	1	19	3	0	0	1	0.5	0	10	0
Lady fingers	1	26	5	0	1	0	0.0	15	50	0
Lorna Doone® shortbread	1	35	5	0	0	2	0.5	0	38	0
Macaroons	1 (2 inch)	101	14	1	1	5	4.5	0	53	1
Mallomars®	1	60	9	½	1	3	1.5	0	20	1
Milano®, milk chocolate	1	57	7	½	1	3	1.5	3	37	0
Molasses	1 medium	65	11	1	1	2	0.5	0	69	0
Mrs. Fields										
rainbow chocolate chip	1 (1.0 oz.)	120	17	1	1	6	3.0	10	115	0
white chunk macadamia	1 (1.1 oz.)	160	21	1 ½	2	8	4.0	15	150	0
Nutter Butter®	1	65	10	½	1	3	1.0	0	53	0
Oatmeal raisin	1 medium	70	11	1	1	3	1.0	5	70	0
Oreo®										
cakesters	1	125	18	1	1	6	1.5	3	125	1
Doublestuf®	1	70	11	1	1	4	1.0	0	53	0
regular	1	53	8	½	0	2	1.0	0	53	0

DESSERTS, SWEETS & TOPPINGS

Cookies

ITEM	AMOUNT	CALORIES	CARBOHYDRATE (g)	CARBOHYDRATE CHOICES	PROTEIN (g)	FAT (g)	SATURATED FAT (g)	CHOLESTEROL (mg)	SODIUM (mg)	FIBER (g)
Oreo® (continued)										
sugar free	1	50	8	½	1	3	1.0	0	55	2
Peanut butter	1 medium	72	9	½	1	4	0.5	0	62	0
Pim's™, soft biscuits	1	50	8	½	0	2	1.0	5	15	0
Sandies®										
pecan shortbread	1	80	9	½	1	5	1.5	0	53	0
simply shortbread	1	80	10	½	1	5	2.0	8	45	0
Shortbread	1 medium	70	8	½	1	4	2.5	12	48	0
SnackWell's®										
chocolate mint	1	50	12	1	1	1	0.0	0	40	0
creme sandwich	1	55	10	½	1	2	0.5	0	45	0
devil's food	1	50	12	1	0	0	0.0	0	25	0
lemon creme	1	43	8	½	0	2	1.0	0	45	1
shortbread	1	43	7	½	1	2	0.5	2	47	1
Social Tea® biscuits	1	20	3	0	0	1	0.0	0	21	0
Sugar	1	72	10	½	1	3	1.0	8	54	0
Sugar wafers	1	18	3	0	0	1	0.5	0	3	0
TimTam™	1	95	12	1	1	5	2.5	0	33	0
Vanilla wafers	1	18	3	0	0	1	0.0	1	14	0
Vienna Fingers®										
reduced fat	1	70	12	1	1	2	1.0	0	58	0
regular	1	75	12	1	1	3	1.0	0	48	0
Frozen Yogurt										
Cherry Garcia®	½ cup	200	37	2 ½	8	3	2.0	20	90	0
Chocolate fudge brownie	½ cup	170	34	2	5	3	0.5	15	95	1
Chocolate/strawberry/vanilla										
fat free	½ cup	90	19	1	3	0	0.0	0	55	0
regular	½ cup	100	17	1	2	3	1.5	10	35	0
Strawberry banana, lowfat	½ cup	160	30	2	3	2	1.0	30	25	1
Ice Cream										
Butter pecan	½ cup	290	20	1	4	21	10.0	70	80	1
Cherry Garcia®	½ cup	240	28	2	4	13	9.0	60	35	0
Chocolate chip cookie dough	½ cup	270	32	2	4	15	10.0	65	85	0
Chocolate fudge brownie	½ cup	260	32	2	5	13	9.0	35	80	2
Chocolate/strawberry/vanilla										
fat free	½ cup	94	20	1	3	0	0.0	0	66	1
light	½ cup	110	17	1	3	3	2.0	15	65	0
light, no added sugar	½ cup	100	13	1	3	3	1.5	10	65	2
premium	½ cup	270	21	1 ½	5	18	11.0	120	70	0
regular	½ cup	140	15	1	3	7	4.5	20	40	0

DESSERTS, SWEETS & TOPPINGS

Ice Cream

ITEM	AMOUNT	CALORIES	CARBOHYDRATE (g)	CARBOHYDRATE CHOICES	PROTEIN (g)	FAT (g)	SATURATED FAT (g)	CHOLESTEROL (mg)	SODIUM (mg)	FIBER (g)
Mint chocolate chip	½ cup	210	19	1	3	13	8.0	45	70	0
Rocky road	½ cup	300	29	2	5	18	9.0	90	75	1
Ice Cream Cones, cone only										
Cake/wafer	1 (0.16 oz.)	15	4	0	0	0	0.0	0	20	0
Sugar	1 (0.46 oz.)	50	10	½	1	1	0.0	0	55	0
Waffle	1 (0.42 oz.)	50	10	½	0	1	0.0	0	25	0
Ice Cream Novelties										
Chocolate éclair bars	1 (3 oz.)	160	21	1 ½	2	8	3.5	5	55	1
Creamsicle®										
original/lowfat	1 (2.3 oz.)	100	20	1	1	2	0.5	0	30	0
sugar free	1 (1.4 oz.)	25	3	0	0	0	0.0	0	5	0
Crunch® bars	1 (2.1 oz.)	200	19	1	1	13	9.0	10	55	0
Dibs®, crunch	26 pieces	340	30	2	2	24	17.0	15	80	0
Dove Bar®	1 (2.6 oz.)	250	24	1 ½	3	17	10.0	30	30	2
Dove® bite size	5 (0.6 oz.)	320	31	2	4	21	13.0	30	35	3
Drumstick® cones	1 (3.3 oz.)	290	33	2	4	16	9.0	15	100	0
Frozen yogurt bars	1 (2.3 oz.)	100	18	1	2	2	1.0	5	25	3
Fruit juice bars	1 (3 oz.)	80	20	1	0	0	0.0	0	0	0
Fudge bars										
Fudgsicle®, no sugar added	1 (1.4 oz.)	40	10	½	2	1	0.0	0	50	2
Fudgsicle®, regular	1 (2.3 oz.)	100	17	1	2	2	1.0	0	80	0
Gelato	½ cup	210	22	1 ½	3	12	8.0	45	70	0
Gelato bars	1 (1.2 oz.)	125	10	½	1	9	6.0	8	9	0
Ice cream sandwiches	1 (3.3 oz.)	180	27	2	3	7	4.0	20	170	1
Italian ice	½ cup	60	20	1	0	0	0.0	0	10	0
Klondike® bars										
Heath®	1 (2.6 oz.)	230	25	1 ½	2	15	11.0	10	80	0
Oreo®	1 (2.6 oz.)	250	29	2	3	15	11.0	10	115	0
original, no sugar added	1 (2.8 oz.)	170	21	1 ½	4	9	8.0	5	65	4
original, regular	1 (3.0 oz.)	250	29	2	3	14	11.0	10	70	0
M&M's® sandwich cookies	1 (2.3 oz.)	220	29	2	3	11	4.5	25	170	1
Popsicle®										
regular	1 (1.9 oz.)	45	11	1	0	0	0.0	0	5	0
sugar free	1 (1.8 oz.)	15	4	0	0	0	0.0	0	0	0
Push-Ups®, sherbet	1 (2.8 oz.)	70	16	1	0	1	0.5	5	15	0
Rice Dream®, nondairy										
carob almond	½ cup	180	26	2	0	10	0.5	0	70	2
cocoa marble fudge	½ cup	170	31	2	0	6	0.5	0	90	1
cookies 'n dream	½ cup	170	27	2	0	8	1.0	0	75	2
Sherbet	½ cup	110	27	2	1	0	0.0	0	25	0

DESSERTS, SWEETS & TOPPINGS
Ice Cream Novelties

ITEM	AMOUNT	CALORIES	CARBOHYDRATE (g)	CARBOHYDRATE CHOICES	PROTEIN (g)	FAT (g)	SATURATED FAT (g)	CHOLESTEROL (mg)	SODIUM (mg)	FIBER (g)
Snickers® bars	1 (1.8 oz.)	180	18	1	3	11	6.0	15	60	1
Snow cones	1 (6.7 oz.)	243	62	4	1	0	0.0	0	42	0
Sorbet	½ cup	120	31	2	0	0	0.0	0	0	0
Soy Dream®, nondairy										
butter pecan	½ cup	190	23	1 ½	1	11	2.0	0	140	1
chocolate fudge brownie	½ cup	170	21	1 ½	0	9	1.5	0	150	1
French vanilla	½ cup	140	17	1	1	8	1.0	0	125	0
Strawberry shortcake bars	1 (2 oz.)	170	21	1 ½	1	9	2.5	5	60	0
Tofutti®	½ cup	210	21	1 ½	2	13	2.0	0	130	0
Other Sweets										
Caramel apples	1 medium	243	54	3 ½	2	4	3.0	3	102	4
Chocolate mousse, w/ 1%, mix	½ cup	128	18	1	4	4	3.5	4	78	0
Crepe Suzette, w/ sauce	1 (2.5 oz.)	171	17	1	4	10	4.0	89	79	0
Custard	½ cup	148	23	1 ½	5	4	2.0	64	118	0
Flan, w/ caramel										
hmde.	½ cup	223	35	2	7	6	3.0	138	81	0
mix	½ cup	150	25	1 ½	4	4	2.5	16	149	0
Gelatin										
regular	½ cup	80	19	1	2	0	0.0	0	90	0
sugar free	½ cup	10	0	0	1	0	0.0	0	60	0
Marshmallows	4 large	100	24	1 ½	0	0	0.0	0	25	0
Pudding										
bread, hmde.	½ cup	199	28	2	6	7	3.5	102	279	1
chocolate, instant, sugar free, w/ skim	½ cup	80	14	1	4	0	0.0	2	361	0
chocolate, instant, w/ 1%	½ cup	155	32	2	5	1	1.0	8	445	0
chocolate, regular, sugar free, w/ skim	½ cup	70	13	1	4	0	0.0	2	161	0
chocolate, regular, w/ 1%	½ cup	145	29	2	5	1	1.0	8	175	0
chocolate, regular, w/ skim	½ cup	132	28	2	4	0	0.0	2	164	0
rice, regular, w/ 1%	½ cup	151	30	2	5	1	1.0	5	159	0
tapioca, w/ 1%	½ cup	150	29	2	5	1	1.0	8	130	0
vanilla, instant, sugar free, w/ skim	½ cup	70	12	1	4	0	0.0	2	351	0
vanilla, instant, w/ 1%	½ cup	145	30	2	5	1	1.0	8	415	0
vanilla, regular, sugar free, w/ skim	½ cup	60	11	1	4	0	0.0	2	166	0
vanilla, regular, w/ 1%	½ cup	135	28	2	5	1	1.0	8	200	0
vanilla, regular, w/ skim	½ cup	122	27	2	4	0	0.0	2	213	0
Pies										
(Based on a 10-inch pie unless indicated.)										
Apple/cherry	1/8 pie	413	60	4	4	19	4.0	0	450	1
Banana cream	1/8 pie	463	55	3 ½	4	26	16.5	25	449	1
Boston cream	1/8 pie	275	40	2 ½	3	11	3.0	38	213	0

DESSERTS, SWEETS & TOPPINGS

Pies

ITEM	AMOUNT	CALORIES	CARBOHYDRATE (g)	CARBOHYDRATE CHOICES	PROTEIN (g)	FAT (g)	SATURATED FAT (g)	CHOLESTEROL (mg)	SODIUM (mg)	FIBER (g)
Chocolate chiffon	1/8 pie	463	55	3 ½	4	26	16.5	25	449	1
Coconut cream	1/8 pie	463	55	3 ½	4	26	16.5	25	449	1
Grasshopper	1/8 pie	450	43	3	6	26	10.5	126	302	1
Hostess® fruit	1 (2 oz.)	230	26	2	2	13	7.5	0	130	0
Key lime	1/8 pie	420	55	3 ½	6	20	12.0	20	200	1
Lemon meringue	1/8 pie	390	65	4	3	14	3.0	15	450	1
Pecan	1/8 pie	550	75	5	7	26	6.0	85	510	2
Pumpkin	1/8 pie	388	59	4	6	15	4.0	56	488	3
Rhubarb	1/8 pie	348	53	3 ½	3	14	4.0	3	217	3
Shoo fly	1/8 pie	453	77	5	5	14	3.0	42	160	1
Strawberry cream	1/8 pie	463	55	3 ½	4	26	16.5	25	449	1
Sweet potato	1/8 pie	390	56	4	7	16	5.0	50	330	2

Syrups & Toppings

ITEM	AMOUNT	CALORIES	CARBOHYDRATE (g)	CARBOHYDRATE CHOICES	PROTEIN (g)	FAT (g)	SATURATED FAT (g)	CHOLESTEROL (mg)	SODIUM (mg)	FIBER (g)
Apple butter	1 T.	31	8	½	0	0	0.0	0	1	0
Artificial sweeteners										
DiabetiSweet®, brown	1 tsp.	10	4	0	0	0	0.0	0	0	0
DiabetiSweet®, white	1 tsp.	9	4	0	0	0	0.0	0	0	0
Equal®	¼ tsp.	0	0	0	0	0	0.0	0	0	0
Splenda®	1 tsp.	0	0	0	0	0	0.0	0	0	0
Stevia®	1 pkt.	0	0	0	0	0	0.0	0	0	0
Stevia in the Raw®	1 tsp.	0	0	0	0	0	0.0	0	0	0
Sugar Twin®, brown/white	1 tsp.	0	0	0	0	0	0.0	0	0	0
Sun Crystals®	½ tsp.	10	2	0	0	0	0.0	0	0	0
SustaBowl™	1 tsp.	6	3	0	0	0	0.0	0	0	0
Sweet 'N Low®	1/10 tsp.	0	0	0	0	0	0.0	0	0	0
Truvia™	¾ tsp.	0	3	0	0	0	0.0	0	0	0
Butterscotch/caramel	2 T.	103	27	2	1	0	0.0	0	143	0
Chocolate syrup										
lite	2 T.	50	12	1	0	0	0.0	0	35	0
regular	2 T.	100	24	1 ½	1	0	0.0	0	25	0
Coffee syrup	2 T.	90	23	1 ½	0	0	0.0	0	20	0
Frosting/icing										
chocolate, reduced sugar	2 T.	120	16	1	0	8	2.0	0	75	1
chocolate, regular	2 T.	140	21	1 ½	0	6	1.5	0	90	0
vanilla, reduced sugar	2 T.	120	18	1	0	7	2.0	0	60	0
vanilla, regular	2 T.	150	24	1 ½	0	6	1.5	0	70	0
Fruit spread	1 T.	40	10	½	0	0	0.0	0	0	0
Grenadine syrup	1 tsp.	18	5	0	0	0	0.0	0	3	0
Honey	1 tsp.	21	6	½	0	0	0.0	0	0	0
Hot fudge										
fat free	2 T.	90	23	1 ½	2	0	0.0	0	90	2

DESSERTS, SWEETS & TOPPINGS
Syrups & Toppings

ITEM	AMOUNT	CALORIES	CARBOHYDRATE (g)	CARBOHYDRATE CHOICES	PROTEIN (g)	FAT (g)	SATURATED FAT (g)	CHOLESTEROL (mg)	SODIUM (mg)	FIBER (g)
Hot fudge *(continued)*										
regular	2 T.	130	22	1 ½	2	5	1.5	0	45	0
Jam/jelly/marmalade	1 T.	50	13	1	0	0	0.0	0	0	0
Maple syrup	1 T.	52	13	1	0	0	0.0	0	2	0
Marshmallow crème	2 T.	110	28	2	0	0	0.0	0	5	0
Pancake syrup										
low calorie	1 T.	25	7	½	0	0	0.0	0	30	0
regular	1 T.	53	13	1	0	0	0.0	0	30	0
Sugar, brown/raw/white	1 tsp.	16	4	0	0	0	0.0	0	0	0
Whipped cream, hmde.	2 T.	52	0	0	0	6	3.5	20	6	0
Whipped toppings										
Cool-Whip®, chocolate/vanilla	2 T.	25	2	0	0	2	1.5	0	0	0
Cool-Whip®, Free™	2 T.	15	3	0	0	0	0.0	0	5	0
Cool-Whip®, Lite®	2 T.	20	3	0	0	1	1.0	0	0	0
Cool-Whip®, regular	2 T.	25	2	0	0	2	1.5	0	0	0
Cool-Whip®, sugar free	2 T.	20	3	0	0	1	1.0	0	0	0
Reddi-Wip®, extra creamy	2 T.	20	0	0	0	2	1.0	5	0	0
Reddi-Wip®, fat free	2 T.	5	1	0	0	0	0.0	0	0	0
Reddi-Wip®, regular	2 T.	15	0	0	0	1	0.5	0	0	0

EGGS, EGG DISHES & EGG SUBSTITUTES
Eggs
Chicken

ITEM	AMOUNT	CALORIES	CARBOHYDRATE (g)	CARBOHYDRATE CHOICES	PROTEIN (g)	FAT (g)	SATURATED FAT (g)	CHOLESTEROL (mg)	SODIUM (mg)	FIBER (g)
boiled/poached	1 large	72	0	0	6	5	1.5	212	70	0
deviled, w/ filling	½	63	0	0	4	5	1.0	122	50	0
Eggland's Best®	1 large	70	0	0	6	4	1.0	170	65	0
fried, w/ ½ tsp. fat	1 large	90	0	0	6	7	2.0	210	94	0
powdered, whites	2 tsp.	10	0	0	3	0	0.0	0	50	0
powdered, whole	2 T.	80	1	0	7	6	2.0	245	75	0
scrambled, w/ 1 tsp. fat	2 large	204	3	0	14	15	4.5	429	342	0
whites	2	33	1	0	7	0	0.0	0	110	0
yolk	1	59	0	0	3	5	1.5	213	7	0
Duck	1	130	1	0	9	10	2.5	619	102	0
Goose	1	266	2	0	20	19	5.0	1227	199	0
Quail	1	14	0	0	1	1	0.5	76	13	0
Turkey	1	135	1	0	11	9	3.0	737	119	0

Egg Dishes

ITEM	AMOUNT	CALORIES	CARBOHYDRATE (g)	CARBOHYDRATE CHOICES	PROTEIN (g)	FAT (g)	SATURATED FAT (g)	CHOLESTEROL (mg)	SODIUM (mg)	FIBER (g)
Frittatas, plain, 10 inch	⅓ pie	233	8	½	16	15	5.0	429	262	0
Omelets										
ham & cheese	1 (2 egg)	369	2	0	27	28	12.5	479	1155	0
ham & cheese	1 (3 egg)	585	3	0	43	45	19.0	725	1944	0

EGGS, EGG DISHES & EGG SUBSTITUTES
Egg Dishes

ITEM	AMOUNT	CALORIES	CARBOHYDRATE (g)	CARBOHYDRATE CHOICES	PROTEIN (g)	FAT (g)	SATURATED FAT (g)	CHOLESTEROL (mg)	SODIUM (mg)	FIBER (g)
Omelets *(continued)*										
vegetable	1 (2 egg)	214	8	½	14	14	4.0	425	180	2
vegetable	1 (3 egg)	332	11	1	21	23	6.0	638	294	2
vegetable, lowfat	1 (6 whites)	159	11	1	23	2	0.5	0	358	2
Quiche										
cheese	4 oz.	336	16	1	10	26	12.5	143	117	0
Lorraine	4 oz.	339	16	1	10	26	12.0	142	142	0
spinach	4 oz.	272	13	1	9	21	9.5	125	89	1
Soufflés										
cheese	1 cup	192	6	½	11	14	5.0	195	274	0
spinach	1 cup	233	8	½	11	18	8.5	160	770	1
Egg Substitutes										
Egg Beaters®	¼ cup	30	1	0	6	0	0.0	0	115	0
Liquid egg whites	¼ cup	29	1	0	6	0	0.0	0	96	0

FAST FOODS & RESTAURANT CHAINS
Arby's®

ITEM	AMOUNT	CALORIES	CARBOHYDRATE (g)	CARBOHYDRATE CHOICES	PROTEIN (g)	FAT (g)	SATURATED FAT (g)	CHOLESTEROL (mg)	SODIUM (mg)	FIBER (g)
Chicken sandwiches										
bacon & Swiss, crispy	1	600	55	3 ½	33	27	7.0	75	1750	4
bacon & Swiss, roast	1	470	43	3	32	19	5.0	65	1310	2
cordon bleu, crispy	1	620	53	3 ½	36	30	6.0	95	2040	3
cordon bleu, roast	1	490	40	2 ½	35	21	5.0	85	1600	2
crispy	1	530	52	3 ½	25	25	4.0	60	1310	4
roast	1	400	40	2 ½	24	16	3.0	50	870	3
roast club	1	500	41	3	31	23	7.0	70	1320	2
Chicken tenders, Prime-Cut™	regular	360	31	2	21	17	2.5	50	1160	2
Chicken tenders, Prime-Cut™	large	610	52	3 ½	35	28	4.0	85	1940	3
Curly fries	medium	600	74	5	6	31	4.0	25	1550	5
Desserts										
apple turnover, w/o icing	1	310	38	2 ½	5	16	7.0	0	190	1
cherry turnover, w/o icing	1	310	37	2 ½	5	16	7.0	0	240	2
chocolate chunk cookies	2	420	54	3 ½	4	21	10.0	30	320	2
Dipping Sauces										
barbeque	1 pkt.	45	11	1	0	0	0.0	0	350	0
Bronco Berry®	1 pkt.	90	22	1 ½	0	0	0.0	0	30	0
Buffalo	1 pkt.	10	1	0	0	1	0.0	0	720	0
honey Dijon mustard	1 pkt.	140	5	0	0	13	2.0	10	130	0
marinara	1 pkt.	35	5	0	1	2	0.0	0	160	1
ranch	1 pkt.	160	2	0	1	16	3.5	30	280	0
Homestyle fries	medium	480	69	4 ½	5	21	3.0	0	1360	5
Jalapeño Bites®	5	300	31	2	5	17	6.0	25	740	2

FAST FOODS & RESTAURANT CHAINS

Arby's®

ITEM	AMOUNT	CALORIES	CARBOHYDRATE (g)	CARBOHYDRATE CHOICES	PROTEIN (g)	FAT (g)	SATURATED FAT (g)	CHOLESTEROL (mg)	SODIUM (mg)	FIBER (g)
Loaded Potato Bites®	5	350	32	2	9	21	6.0	40	810	3
Market Fresh® farmhouse chopped salads										
chicken, crispy	1	430	30	2	27	24	8.0	65	1150	4
chicken, roast	1	250	11	1	23	13	7.0	60	680	3
side	1	70	4	0	4	5	3.0	15	100	1
turkey & ham	1	250	10	½	23	14	7.0	60	910	3
Market Fresh® sandwiches										
pecan chicken salad	1	750	85	5 ½	29	34	4.5	55	1350	4
Reuben	1	700	64	4	38	32	9.0	65	1870	4
roast beef & Swiss	1	770	78	5	38	35	10.0	85	1680	5
roast ham & Swiss	1	710	78	5	36	30	8.0	75	2010	5
roast turkey & Swiss	1	710	78	5	39	28	7.0	75	1780	5
roast turkey ranch & bacon	1	810	78	5	46	36	10.0	95	2270	5
ultimate BLT	1	820	78	5	32	44	9.0	45	1690	5
Mozzarella sticks	4	440	39	2 ½	21	23	9.0	5	1190	2
Potato cakes	2	260	28	2	2	15	2.0	0	400	2
Roast beef sandwiches										
All-American Roastburger®	1	390	44	3	20	15	5.0	45	1730	2
Arby's® melt	1	370	40	2 ½	23	13	4.0	50	1150	2
Bacon Cheddar Roastburger®	1	420	42	3	26	16	8.0	60	1840	2
beef'n cheddar	regular	420	43	3	23	18	5.0	50	1260	2
ham & Swiss melt	1	300	37	2 ½	18	8	3.5	35	1070	2
original	regular	340	38	2 ½	23	11	4.0	45	970	2
original	large	560	47	3	45	22	8.0	110	1870	3
Salad dressings										
balsamic vinaigrette	1 pkt.	130	5	0	0	12	2.0	0	470	0
buttermilk ranch	1 pkt.	210	2	0	1	23	3.5	10	380	0
Dijon honey mustard	1 pkt.	180	8	½	0	16	2.5	15	260	0
Shakes										
chocolate	small	450	75	5	12	12	8.0	45	350	1
jamocha	small	440	75	5	11	12	8.0	45	350	1
vanilla	small	380	60	4	11	12	8.0	45	310	0
Toasted sandwiches										
classic Italian	1	590	57	4	24	30	8.0	55	1870	3
French dip & Swiss	1	500	61	4	29	15	6.0	60	2220	2
Philly beef	1	560	56	4	28	25	7.0	65	1490	3
turkey bacon club	1	560	56	4	32	23	6.0	60	1710	3

Boston Market®

Desserts

ITEM	AMOUNT	CALORIES	CARBOHYDRATE (g)	CARBOHYDRATE CHOICES	PROTEIN (g)	FAT (g)	SATURATED FAT (g)	CHOLESTEROL (mg)	SODIUM (mg)	FIBER (g)
apple pie	1	580	74	5	4	30	13.0	0	690	3
chocolate cake	1	580	67	4 ½	5	34	11.0	45	360	3

FAST FOODS & RESTAURANT CHAINS
Boston Market®

ITEM	AMOUNT	CALORIES	CARBOHYDRATE (g)	CARBOHYDRATE CHOICES	PROTEIN (g)	FAT (g)	SATURATED FAT (g)	CHOLESTEROL (mg)	SODIUM (mg)	FIBER (g)
Desserts *(continued)*										
chocolate chip fudge brownie	1	320	49	3	5	13	3.0	50	220	3
cornbread	1	200	34	2	3	6	2.0	10	300	1
Nestlé® Toll House® chocolate chip cookie	1	370	50	3	3	19	10.0	20	340	1
pecan pie	1	640	74	5	7	36	11.0	115	340	2
pumpkin pie	1	430	57	4	6	22	10.0	45	380	2
Individual plates, w/o sides										
BBQ chicken slider	1 order	240	36	2 ½	11	6	2.0	30	720	0
beef brisket	regular	230	0	0	28	13	3.5	95	570	0
beef brisket	large	400	1	0	48	23	6.0	165	990	0
meatloaf	regular	480	25	1 ½	28	30	13.0	145	1090	6
meatloaf	large	720	38	2	42	45	20.0	218	1635	9
meatloaf slider	1 order	290	34	2	13	13	5.0	40	670	2
pastry top chicken pot pie	1 order	810	60	4	33	48	24.0	140	1280	4
pastry top turkey pot pie	1 order	790	60	4	34	46	23.0	90	1220	4
roasted turkey breast	regular	180	0	0	38	3	1.0	70	620	0
roasted turkey breast	large	260	0	0	54	5	2.0	100	870	0
turkey slider	1 order	280	24	1 ½	14	15	3.5	30	510	0
Rotisserie chicken, w/o sides										
¼ chicken, white meat	1 order	320	0	0	52	12	4.0	200	900	0
¼ chicken, white meat, w/o skin	1 order	240	1	0	50	4	1.0	180	890	0
1 thigh & 1 drumstick	1 order	290	0	0	37	17	5.0	210	950	0
3 pc. dark (2 thighs & drumstick)	1 order	490	0	0	60	29	8.0	335	1600	0
3 pc. dark, individual meal	1 order	390	1	0	51	22	6.0	290	1270	0
3 pc. dk., w/o skin (2 thighs & drmstk)	1 order	350	0	0	52	15	4.5	280	1210	0
3 pc. dk., w/o skin (thigh & 2 drmstk)	1 order	290	0	0	45	11	3.5	240	1010	0
half chicken	1 order	610	1	0	89	29	9.0	405	1860	0
Salads, w/ dressing										
Asian	1	570	33	2	40	31	5.0	100	1280	5
Caesar	1	500	25	1 ½	14	39	9.0	30	1190	3
Caesar, w/ chicken	1	650	26	2	45	42	10.0	130	1680	3
Mediterranean	1	670	27	2	40	45	10.0	125	1380	3
Southwest Santa Fe	1	690	41	2 ½	41	42	9.0	125	1560	5
Sandwiches										
all white rotisserie chicken salad	1	1040	88	5 ½	41	60	9.0	110	1780	11
brisket & Swiss dip	1	840	62	4	46	45	12.0	135	1660	3
meatloaf & cheddar	1	940	96	6	46	40	18.0	170	2430	10
roasted turkey & Swiss carver	1	790	66	4 ½	50	35	9.0	95	1810	3
rotisserie chicken carver	1	840	66	4 ½	57	37	9.0	165	2080	3
rotisserie chicken pesto	1	1030	89	5 ½	61	52	9.0	150	2290	11
turkey BLT	1	1030	89	5 ½	48	57	11.0	90	2190	11

FAST FOODS & RESTAURANT CHAINS
Boston Market®

ITEM	AMOUNT	CALORIES	CARBOHYDRATE (g)	CARBOHYDRATE CHOICES	PROTEIN (g)	FAT (g)	SATURATED FAT (g)	CHOLESTEROL (mg)	SODIUM (mg)	FIBER (g)
Sides										
cinnamon apples	1 order	210	47	3	0	3	0.0	0	15	3
coleslaw	1 order	410	13	1	2	40	6.0	15	410	2
garlic dill new potatoes	1 order	140	24	1 ½	3	3	1.0	0	120	3
garlic lemon savoy spinach	1 order	140	9	½	6	10	6.0	25	440	5
green beans	1 order	60	7	½	2	4	1.5	0	180	3
loaded mashed potatoes	1 order	310	33	2	8	16	8.0	45	850	3
macaroni & cheese	1 order	140	35	2	11	11	7.0	30	1100	2
mashed potatoes	1 order	270	36	2 ½	5	11	5.0	25	820	4
Mediterranean green beans	1 order	120	10	½	3	9	2.5	0	220	4
squash casserole	1 order	270	20	1	9	17	7.0	30	1120	3
steamed vegetables	1 order	60	8	½	2	2	0.0	0	40	3
sweet corn	1 order	170	37	2 ½	6	4	1.0	0	95	2
sweet potato casserole	1 order	460	77	5	4	16	4.5	5	270	3
vegetable stuffing	1 order	190	25	1 ½	3	8	1.0	0	580	2
Soups										
broccoli cheese	1 order	480	25	1 ½	22	33	21.0	95	1490	4
chicken noodle	1 order	250	23	1 ½	22	8	2.5	95	1420	2
chicken tortilla, w/o toppings	1 order	160	13	1	10	8	1.5	45	1690	2
Burger King®										
BK Breakfast Bowl™	1	540	17	1	24	42	13.0	375	1020	n/a
BK Fish Filet® sandwich, w/ tartar sauce	1	640	66	4 ½	23	32	5.0	45	1370	n/a
BK Veggie® burger, w/o mayo.	1	320	43	3	22	7	1.0	0	960	n/a
Chicken sandwiches										
original, w/ mayo	1	630	46	3	24	39	7.0	65	1390	n/a
Spicy Chick'n Crisp®, w/ mayo.	1	460	35	2	13	30	5.0	30	810	n/a
Tender Grill®, w/ mayo	1	470	40	2 ½	55	18	7.0	85	1100	n/a
Tendercrisp® w/ mayo	1	800	68	4 ½	32	46	8.0	70	1640	n/a
Chicken Tenders®	5	230	16	1	11	13	2.5	35	380	n/a
Croissan'wich®										
egg & cheese	1	320	26	2	11	16	7.0	180	690	n/a
egg & cheese, w/ bacon	1	360	26	2	14	19	8.0	190	840	n/a
Dutch apple pie	1	320	47	3	2	13	5.0	0	290	n/a
French fries										
small, salted	1 order	340	44	3	4	17	3.5	0	530	n/a
small, unsalted	1 order	340	44	3	4	17	3.5	0	380	n/a
medium, salted	1 order	440	56	4	5	22	4.5	0	670	n/a
large, salted	1 order	540	69	4 ½	6	27	6.0	0	830	n/a
French toast sticks w/ syrup	3 pieces	350	59	4	3	11	2.0	0	280	n/a
Hamburgers										
cheeseburger	1	300	28	2	16	14	6.0	45	710	n/a

FAST FOODS & RESTAURANT CHAINS

Burger King®

ITEM	AMOUNT	CALORIES	CARBOHYDRATE (g)	CARBOHYDRATE CHOICES	PROTEIN (g)	FAT (g)	SATURATED FAT (g)	CHOLESTEROL (mg)	SODIUM (mg)	FIBER (g)
Hamburgers *(continued)*										
double cheeseburger	1	450	29	2	27	26	12.0	95	960	n/a
hamburger	1	260	27	2	13	10	4.0	35	490	n/a
Steakhouse XT™ burger	1	770	53	3 ½	36	46	17.0	115	1380	n/a
Hamburgers, Whopper®										
Double Whopper®	1	900	51	3 ½	47	57	19.0	140	980	n/a
w/o mayo.	1	740	51	3 ½	47	39	16.0	130	840	n/a
Double Whopper®, w/ cheese	1	990	53	3 ½	52	65	24.0	160	1410	n/a
w/o mayo.	1	830	53	3 ½	52	47	21.0	150	1270	n/a
Whopper®	1	670	51	3 ½	28	40	11.0	75	980	n/a
w/o mayo.	1	510	51	3 ½	28	22	9.0	65	840	n/a
Whopper®, w/ cheese	1	710	52	3 ½	30	43	14.0	85	1190	n/a
w/o mayo.	1	560	52	3 ½	30	26	11.0	75	1050	n/a
Whopper Jr®	1	340	29	2	14	19	5.0	40	530	n/a
w/o mayo.	1	260	29	2	13	10	4.0	35	460	n/a
Whopper Jr®, w/ cheese	1	390	29	2	16	23	8.0	55	740	n/a
w/o mayo.	1	310	29	2	16	14	6.0	45	670	n/a
Hash brown rounds	small	250	24	1 ½	2	16	3.5	0	410	n/a
Onion rings										
value	1 order	150	7	½	2	8	1.5	0	230	n/a
small	1 order	310	36	2 ½	4	17	3.0	0	490	n/a
medium	1 order	450	52	3 ½	6	24	4.0	0	700	n/a
Salads, w/ dressing										
side garden	1	330	18	1	6	26	6.0	30	770	n/a
Tendercrisp® chicken garden	1	670	38	2 ½	29	45	9.0	85	1740	n/a
Tendergrill® chicken garden	1	490	20	1	36	30	7.0	110	1600	n/a
Shakes										
chocolate	small	440	78	5	9	11	8.0	40	360	n/a
chocolate	medium	650	119	8	12	16	12.0	50	530	n/a
strawberry	small	430	77	5	8	11	8.0	40	290	n/a
strawberry	medium	630	116	8	11	15	11.0	50	400	n/a
vanilla	small	370	60	4	9	12	9.0	40	310	n/a
vanilla	medium	520	84	5 ½	12	16	12.0	55	420	n/a
Value meals, w/ medium soda & medium fries										
BK® chicken fries, 9 piece	1 meal	1110	157	10 ½	26	44	8.5	40	1900	n/a
Double Whopper®	1 meal	1630	184	12	52	79	23.5	140	1660	n/a
Steakhouse XT™ burger	1 meal	1500	186	12 ½	41	68	21.5	115	2060	n/a
Tendercrisp® chicken sandwich	1 meal	1530	201	13 ½	37	68	12.5	70	2320	n/a
Whopper®	1 meal	1400	184	12	33	62	15.5	75	1660	n/a
Whopper Jr.®	1 meal	1070	162	11	19	41	9.5	40	1210	n/a

Chili's®

ITEM	AMOUNT	CALORIES	CARBOHYDRATE (g)	CARBOHYDRATE CHOICES	PROTEIN (g)	FAT (g)	SATURATED FAT (g)	CHOLESTEROL (mg)	SODIUM (mg)	FIBER (g)
Appetizers, as served										
boneless Buffalo wings, w/ blue cheese	1 order	1490	94	6	76	88	16.0	n/a	4590	2
classic nachos, beef	8 piece	1170	59	3 ½	67	74	38.0	n/a	2430	8
crispy onion string & jalapeño stack, w/ ranch	1 order	1050	71	5	12	81	18.0	n/a	2230	4
hot spinach & artichoke dip, w/ chips	1 order	1610	139	9	33	103	42.0	n/a	1610	14
Southwestern eggrolls, w/ avocado ranch	1 order	780	81	5	24	41	10.0	n/a	1830	7
tostada chips, w/ salsa	1 order	1020	125	8	12	51	10.0	n/a	1210	11
Wings Over Buffalo®, w/ blue cheese	1 order	690	7	½	41	53	11.0	n/a	2100	1
Big Mouth® burgers, w/ fries										
Big Mouth® bites, w/ jalapeño ranch	1 order	2120	163	10 ½	66	133	38.0	n/a	4810	7
classic bacon burger	1 order	1570	125	8	61	90	29.0	n/a	3690	9
mushroom-Swiss	1 order	1540	126	8	59	88	28.0	n/a	3710	10
Oldtimer®	1 order	1310	128	8	51	65	20.0	n/a	3230	10
Chicken/Fish dinners, as served										
Crispy Chicken Crispers®, w/o sauce	1 order	1210	125	8	52	57	10.0	n/a	2670	13
fried shrimp, w/ cocktail sauce	1 order	990	108	7	26	52	11.0	n/a	3650	9
grilled salmon, w/ garlic & herbs	1 order	580	38	2	49	28	10.0	n/a	1660	5
Margarita grilled chicken	1 order	550	62	4	46	14	4.0	n/a	1870	8
Monterey Chicken®	1 order	860	51	3	64	46	19.0	n/a	2860	8
Desserts										
brownie sundae	1	1290	195	13	14	61	30.0	n/a	930	8
cheesecake	1 piece	710	68	4 ½	12	42	26.0	n/a	460	0
molten chocolate cake, w/ ice cream	1	1020	144	9 ½	11	46	27.0	n/a	710	5
Fajita sides										
fajita condiments	1 order	230	7	½	10	19	10.0	n/a	490	3
flour tortillas	3	390	63	4	10	10	3.0	n/a	1040	3
Fajitas										
beef	1 order	390	27	1 ½	37	14	5.0	n/a	1950	7
chicken	1 order	360	24	1	44	10	3.0	n/a	1330	7
trio	1 order	530	30	2	56	20	7.0	n/a	2340	8
Quesadillas, as served										
bacon ranch chicken	1 order	1650	96	6	78	107	39.0	n/a	3450	5
bacon ranch steak	1 order	1680	98	6	74	111	41.0	n/a	3940	5
Ribs, as served										
Memphis dry rub, full rack	1 order	1990	137	8 ½	119	111	37.0	n/a	6180	21
original, full rack	1 order	2170	137	8 ½	133	123	44.0	n/a	6510	20
original, half rack	1 order	1140	75	4 ½	69	63	23.0	n/a	3800	9

FAST FOODS & RESTAURANT CHAINS

Chili's®

ITEM	AMOUNT	CALORIES	CARBOHYDRATE (g)	CARBOHYDRATE CHOICES	PROTEIN (g)	FAT (g)	SATURATED FAT (g)	CHOLESTEROL (mg)	SODIUM (mg)	FIBER (g)
Ribs *(continued)*										
Shiner Bock® BBQ, full rack	1 order	2310	168	10 ½	134	123	44.0	n/a	6340	20
Salads, w/ dressing										
boneless Buffalo chicken	1 order	990	48	3	46	68	14.0	n/a	4310	8
Caribbean, w/ grilled chicken	1 order	610	65	4	33	25	4.0	n/a	800	6
Caribbean, w/ grilled shrimp	1 order	620	66	4	19	31	6.0	n/a	1060	6
chicken Caesar	1 order	650	26	1 ½	40	44	8.0	n/a	1130	5
house, w/o dressing	1 order	180	15	1	10	11	6.0	n/a	290	2
quesadilla explosion	1 order	1400	90	5 ½	65	89	28.0	n/a	2360	9
Sandwiches, w/ fries (unless indicated)										
BBQ pulled pork	1 order	1670	172	11	54	85	16.0	n/a	4240	13
Buffalo chicken ranch	1 order	1410	143	9	52	68	12.0	n/a	3940	12
grilled chicken, w/ steamed broccoli	1 order	610	78	5	43	13	5.0	n/a	1320	8
smoked turkey	1 order	1340	138	9	41	64	17.0	n/a	3140	11
Sides										
black beans	1 side	100	18	1	6	1	0.0	n/a	620	5
cinnamon apples	1 side	280	48	3	0	11	2.0	n/a	130	9
cole slaw	1 side	240	15	1	1	20	4.0	n/a	490	2
corn on the cob, w/ butter	1 side	200	32	2	5	7	1.0	n/a	420	3
guacamole	1 side	45	3	0	1	4	0.0	n/a	140	2
homestyle fries	1 side	380	61	4	4	13	3.0	n/a	1210	6
loaded mashed potatoes	1 side	390	28	2	13	25	9.0	n/a	1170	3
rice	1 side	240	41	3	4	6	1.0	n/a	410	1
seasonal veggies	1 side	80	7	½	3	6	3.0	n/a	490	3
Soups/chili										
broccoli cheese	1 cup	110	8	½	5	7	4.0	n/a	600	1
chicken enchilada	1 cup	200	11	1	11	13	5.0	n/a	820	1
loaded baked potato	1 cup	210	11	½	8	15	9.0	n/a	590	8
Terlingua chili w/ toppings	1 cup	180	9	½	14	10	5.0	n/a	580	3
Steak dinners, as served										
classic sirloin	1 order	1010	59	3 ½	62	60	24.0	n/a	3370	7
classic sirloin, guiltless grill	1 order	370	20	1	53	9	4.0	n/a	3680	6
country-fried	1 order	1270	120	7 ½	41	71	14.0	n/a	3700	9
flame grilled ribeye	1 order	1570	57	3 ½	78	116	50.0	n/a	3560	7
Tacos, as served										
chicken club	1 order	1260	120	7 ½	59	60	18.0	n/a	4320	11
crispy chicken	1 order	1630	171	11	63	78	22.0	n/a	4320	13
crispy shrimp	1 order	1500	174	11	51	68	20.0	n/a	4760	22
Chipotle®										
Barbacoa	4 oz.	170	2	0	24	7	2.5	60	510	0
Black beans	4 oz.	120	23	1	7	1	0.0	0	250	11

FAST FOODS & RESTAURANT CHAINS

Chipotle®

ITEM	AMOUNT	CALORIES	CARBOHYDRATE (g)	CARBOHYDRATE CHOICES	PROTEIN (g)	FAT (g)	SATURATED FAT (g)	CHOLESTEROL (mg)	SODIUM (mg)	FIBER (g)
Carnitas	4 oz.	190	1	0	27	8	2.5	70	540	0
Cheese	1 oz.	100	0	0	8	9	5.0	30	180	0
Chicken	4 oz.	190	1	0	32	7	2.0	115	370	0
Chips	4 oz.	570	73	4 ½	8	27	3.5	0	420	8
Cilantro-lime rice	3 oz.	130	23	1 ½	2	3	0.5	0	150	0
Corn salsa	3.5 oz.	80	15	1	3	2	0.0	0	410	3
Crispy taco shell	1	60	9	½	0	2	0.5	0	10	1
Fajita vegetables	2.5 oz.	20	4	0	1	1	0.0	0	170	1
Flour tortilla, burrito	1	290	44	3	7	9	3.0	0	670	2
Flour tortilla, taco	1	90	13	1	2	3	1.0	0	200	1
Green tomatillo salsa	2 fl. oz.	15	3	0	1	0	0.0	0	230	1
Guacamole	3.5 oz.	150	8	0	2	13	2.0	0	190	6
Pinto beans	4 oz.	120	22	1	7	1	0.0	5	330	10
Red tomatillo salsa	2 fl. oz.	40	8	½	2	1	0.0	0	510	4
Romaine lettuce, salad	2.5 oz.	10	2	0	1	0	0.0	0	5	1
Romaine lettuce, tacos	1 oz.	5	1	0	0	0	0.0	0	0	1
Sour cream	2 oz.	120	2	0	2	10	7.0	40	30	0
Steak	4 oz.	190	2	0	30	7	2.0	65	320	0
Tomato salsa	3.5 oz.	20	4	0	1	0	0.0	0	470	0
Vinaigrette	2 fl. oz.	260	12	1	0	25	4.0	0	700	1

Dairy Queen®

ITEM	AMOUNT	CALORIES	CARBOHYDRATE (g)	CARBOHYDRATE CHOICES	PROTEIN (g)	FAT (g)	SATURATED FAT (g)	CHOLESTEROL (mg)	SODIUM (mg)	FIBER (g)
Banana split	1	520	94	6	9	14	10.0	30	160	4
Blizzard®, chocolate chip cookie dough										
small	1	710	104	7	13	28	16.0	55	400	1
medium	1	1020	148	10	17	40	24.0	75	580	2
Blizzard®, Oreo Cookies®										
small	1	550	81	5 ½	12	20	10.0	40	410	1
medium	1	680	100	6 ½	14	25	12.0	50	530	1
Buster Bar®	1	480	45	3	11	31	15.0	20	220	2
Chicken sandwiches										
crispy	1	560	47	3	20	27	3.5	35	1010	3
grilled	1	370	32	2	24	16	2.5	55	810	1
Chicken Strip Basket®, w/ gravy	4 piece	1160	120	7 ½	40	47	7.0	70	2960	9
Chili 'n' cheese dog	1	380	23	1 ½	16	24	11.0	55	980	1
Chocolate Dilly® bar	1	240	24	1 ½	4	15	9.0	15	70	1
Dipped cones										
chocolate, w/ vanilla soft serve	small	330	42	3	6	15	12.0	25	110	0
chocolate, w/ vanilla soft serve	medium	470	61	4	9	22	18.0	30	150	1
DQ® cakes, 10 inch										
Chocolate Xtreme Blizzard®	1/12 cake	630	84	5 ½	10	29	21.0	35	320	2
Oreo Blizzard® cake	1/12 cake	540	76	5	9	23	15.0	30	320	1

FAST FOODS & RESTAURANT CHAINS

Dairy Queen®

ITEM	AMOUNT	CALORIES	CARBOHYDRATE (g)	CARBOHYDRATE CHOICES	PROTEIN (g)	FAT (g)	SATURATED FAT (g)	CHOLESTEROL (mg)	SODIUM (mg)	FIBER (g)
DQ® fudge bar, no sugar added	1	50	13	½	4	0	0.0	0	70	6
DQ Homestyle® burgers										
¼ lb. Flame Thrower Grillburger®	1	740	41	3	30	51	15.0	100	1200	2
bacon double cheeseburger	1	730	35	2	41	41	21.0	150	1550	1
cheeseburger	1	400	34	2	19	18	9.0	65	920	1
double cheeseburger	1	640	34	2	34	34	18.0	125	1230	1
DQ® ice cream sandwich	1	190	31	2	4	5	3.0	10	135	1
DQ® soft serve, cone, chocolate										
small	1	240	37	2 ½	6	7	5.0	20	115	0
medium	1	340	54	3 ½	9	10	7.0	30	160	0
DQ® soft serve, cone, vanilla										
small	1	330	53	3 ½	9	10	6.0	30	140	0
medium	1	470	74	5	12	14	9.0	45	200	0
DQ® vanilla orange bar, no sugar added	1	60	18	1	2	0	0.0	0	40	6
French fries	regular	310	43	3	4	13	2.0	0	640	3
Hot dog	1	290	22	1 ½	11	17	7.0	35	900	1
Malts, chocolate										
small	1	600	92	6	14	22	15.0	50	250	1
medium	1	800	130	8 ½	17	27	17.0	60	340	1
MooLattes®										
cappuccino	small	450	65	4	8	16	12.0	30	150	0
French vanilla	small	500	80	5	8	15	12.0	30	150	0
mocha	small	500	74	5	8	19	13.0	30	170	0
Onion rings	1 order	360	47	3	6	16	2.0	0	840	2
Oreo Brownie Earthquake®	1	770	119	8	11	27	16.0	60	400	1
Peanut Buster® parfait	1	710	96	6 ½	17	31	18.0	35	350	3
Shakes, chocolate										
small	1	540	80	5	12	21	15.0	45	220	1
medium	1	710	112	7 ½	15	26	17.0	60	280	1
Starkiss Bar®	1	80	21	1 ½	0	0	0.0	0	10	0
Sundae, caramel										
small	1	300	50	3	6	8	5.0	25	140	0
medium	1	430	74	5	9	11	7.0	35	210	0
Sundae, chocolate										
small	1	280	48	3	6	8	4.5	25	115	1
medium	1	400	70	4 ½	8	12	7.0	30	170	1

Denny's®

Appetizers *(Listed w/o condiments or bread.)*

ITEM	AMOUNT	CALORIES	CARBOHYDRATE (g)	CARBOHYDRATE CHOICES	PROTEIN (g)	FAT (g)	SATURATED FAT (g)	CHOLESTEROL (mg)	SODIUM (mg)	FIBER (g)
basket of puppies, w/o syrup	10 pieces	510	100	6 ½	11	11	2.0	0	1640	4
cheese burger flatbread	1 (11 oz.)	890	53	3	38	54	22.0	102	1620	6
cheese quesadilla	1 (8 oz.)	690	48	3	25	42	21.0	75	1300	6

FAST FOODS & RESTAURANT CHAINS
Denny's®

ITEM	AMOUNT	CALORIES	CARBOHYDRATE (g)	CARBOHYDRATE CHOICES	PROTEIN (g)	FAT (g)	SATURATED FAT (g)	CHOLESTEROL (mg)	SODIUM (mg)	FIBER (g)
Appetizers *(continued)*										
chicken strips w/ Buffalo sauce	1 (13 oz.)	720	52	3 ½	57	32	0.0	115	2780	0
chicken wings w/ Buffalo sauce	1 (8 oz.)	330	3	0	34	20	5.0	185	1860	1
mozzarella cheese sticks	1 (8 oz.)	560	58	4	38	20	17.0	185	2480	2
Sampler®	1 (17 oz.)	1380	139	9	53	71	6.0	80	3710	6
smothered cheese fries	1 (10 oz.)	860	75	5	21	53	17.0	65	990	7
three-dip & chips	1 (12 oz.)	560	72	4 ½	19	25	11.0	70	1430	7
zesty nachos	1 (22 oz.)	1340	140	9	62	61	29.0	210	2800	12
Breakfast *(Listed w/o toppings, bread or sides.)*										
All-American Slam®	1 (10 oz.)	800	5	0	40	68	25.0	775	1410	1
bacon	4 strips	140	1	0	9	11	4.0	30	467	0
bagel, w/ cream cheese	1 (6 oz.)	428	48	3	12	11	7.0	35	560	2
Belgian Waffle Slam®	1 (13 oz.)	820	32	2	30	64	27.0	700	1270	2
buttermilk pancakes	2 cakes	330	67	4 ½	8	4	0.5	0	1170	2
English muffin, dry	1 (2 oz.)	130	25	1 ½	4	1	0.0	0	250	1
Fit Slam®	1 (15 oz.)	390	46	3	27	12	4.0	40	850	5
French Toast Slam®	1 (15 oz.)	780	35	2	30	58	21.0	635	1360	2
grits, w/ margarine	1 (12 oz.)	220	44	3	5	3	1.0	0	15	3
ham, grilled	3 oz. slice	120	8	½	14	5	4.0	45	710	0
hash browns	1 (4 oz.)	210	26	2	2	12	2.5	0	650	2
Lumberjack Slam®	1 (17 oz.)	960	80	5	44	50	8.0	550	2820	4
maple-flavored syrup	3 T.	143	36	2 ½	0	0	0.0	0	26	0
maple-flavored syrup, sugar-free	3 T.	23	9	½	0	0	0.0	0	71	0
margarine, whipped	1 tsp.	15	0	0	0	2	0.0	0	10	0
meat lover's scramble	1 (21 oz.)	1140	94	6	49	63	27.0	565	3410	5
Moons Over My Hammy®	1 (13 oz.)	760	51	3 ½	44	41	15.0	530	2320	2
Moons Over My Hammy® Omelette™	1 (16 oz.)	770	31	2	42	53	18.0	790	2590	2
one egg	1 (2 oz.)	120	0	0	6	10	3.0	210	120	0
sausage	4 links	370	4	0	9	34	13.0	70	660	0
The Grand Slamwich® w/ hash browns	1 (21 oz.)	1520	97	6	53	101	44.0	540	3550	5
veggie-cheese omelette	1 (13 oz.)	460	9	½	28	33	12.0	740	680	2
Condiments										
BBQ sauce, sweet & spicy	1.5 oz.	110	30	2	0	0	0.0	0	470	0
pico de gallo	3 oz.	21	5	0	1	0	0.0	0	125	1
sour cream	1.5 oz.	91	2	0	1	9	0.0	19	23	0
Dessert toppings										
cherry	2 oz.	57	14	1	0	0	0.0	0	3	0
fudge	1.5 oz.	150	23	1 ½	1	6	6.0	0	65	1
strawberry	2 oz.	60	14	1	0	0	0.0	0	10	1
whipped cream	2 T.	23	2	0	0	2	0.0	7	3	0

FAST FOODS & RESTAURANT CHAINS

Denny's®

ITEM	AMOUNT	CALORIES	CARBOHYDRATE (g)	CARBOHYDRATE CHOICES	PROTEIN (g)	FAT (g)	SATURATED FAT (g)	CHOLESTEROL (mg)	SODIUM (mg)	FIBER (g)
Desserts										
apple pie	1 (7 oz.)	480	67	4 ½	4	22	9.0	0	580	3
caramel apple crisp	1 (13 oz.)	740	134	9	7	21	9.0	35	570	5
cheesecake	1 (5 oz.)	510	43	3	9	34	20.0	160	370	1
chocolate peanut butter silk pie	1 (6 oz.)	680	59	4	8	47	24.0	70	400	4
coconut cream pie	1 (7 oz.)	630	65	4	6	39	24.0	0	370	1
double scoop/sundae	1 (5 oz.)	370	50	3	5	18	12.0	50	135	1
floats, root beer/cola	1 (16 oz.)	430	69	4 ½	6	17	9.0	65	120	0
Hershey's® chocolate cake	1 (5 oz.)	580	75	5	6	28	15.0	40	400	2
key lime pie	1 (7 oz.)	560	87	6	9	20	8.0	25	320	0
milkshake	1 (12 oz.)	640	80	5	13	31	17.0	120	220	1
Oreo® Blender Blaster™	1 (14 oz.)	890	113	7 ½	15	44	20.0	105	590	3
single scoop/sundae	1 (4 oz.)	300	36	2 ½	4	16	11.0	40	90	1
Entrées *(Listed w/o sides, bread or condiments unless indicated.)*										
chicken strips w/ bread	10 oz.	760	84	5 ½	44	29	6.0	100	1830	3
country fried steak, w/ gravy	1 (15 oz.)	1170	74	5	55	74	25.0	75	2920	6
fish & chips	1 (23 oz.)	1530	145	9	41	90	15.0	130	2430	10
lemon pepper grilled tilapia, w/ bread	1 (15 oz.)	800	59	4	58	35	15.0	155	1740	3
mushroom Swiss chopped steak, w/ bread	1 (16 oz.)	1080	34	2	58	75	30.0	165	2240	2
prime rib & chicken sizzlin' skillet	1 (20 oz.)	940	67	4 ½	69	43	16.0	170	2400	2
T-bone steak, w/ bread	1 (12 oz.)	820	24	1 ½	101	35	12.0	180	1420	1
Salad dressings										
bleu cheese	1 oz.	110	1	0	1	11	3.0	20	220	0
Caesar	1 oz.	100	0	0	1	10	0.0	5	300	0
fat free Italian	1 oz.	9	3	0	0	0	0.0	0	367	0
fat free ranch	1 oz.	25	5	0	0	0	0.0	0	230	0
French	1 oz.	74	8	½	0	5	0.0	7	248	0
ranch	1 oz.	130	0	0	0	14	3.0	5	200	0
thousand island	1 oz.	107	5	0	0	11	2.0	15	170	0
Salads *(Listed w/o salad dressing or bread unless indicated.)*										
chicken deluxe, fried strips	1 (18 oz.)	590	43	3	42	29	5.0	90	1180	4
chicken deluxe, grilled	1 (17 oz.)	340	13	1	44	13	6.0	110	530	4
cranberry apple chicken	1 (13 oz.)	370	32	2	36	12	3.0	90	610	3
garden	1 (7 oz.)	120	7	½	7	7	5.0	20	150	2
Sandwiches *(Listed w/o French fries, sides or condiments unless indicated.)*										
bacon cheddar burger	1 (15 oz.)	880	45	3	52	49	22.0	160	1810	4
BLT	1 (7 oz.)	520	35	2	15	35	8.0	35	620	2
chicken ranch melt	1 (13 oz.)	910	76	5	36	52	14.0	85	2860	3
classic burger, w/fries	1 (19 oz.)	1190	101	7	56	62	21.0	110	1190	0
classic cheeseburger	1 (15 oz.)	820	47	3	47	44	21.0	130	1450	4
club	1 (11 oz.)	630	55	3 ½	26	33	5.0	50	1530	4

FAST FOODS & RESTAURANT CHAINS
Denny's®

ITEM	AMOUNT	CALORIES	CARBOHYDRATE (g)	CARBOHYDRATE CHOICES	PROTEIN (g)	FAT (g)	SATURATED FAT (g)	CHOLESTEROL (mg)	SODIUM (mg)	FIBER (g)
Sandwiches (continued)										
hickory grilled chicken	1 (15 oz.)	900	67	4	50	47	12.0	115	1370	5
mushroom Swiss burger	1 (18 oz.)	860	51	3	49	48	21.0	130	1750	5
prime rib Philly melt	1 (13 oz.)	670	52	3 ½	35	36	11.0	75	1770	3
spicy Buffalo chicken melt	1 (15 oz.)	860	76	5	32	48	12.0	70	3760	3
The Super Bird®	1 (11 oz.)	610	54	3 ½	34	29	9.0	55	2320	2
veggie burger	1 (15 oz.)	540	76	4 ½	31	13	5.0	20	1340	11
Western burger	1 (16 oz.)	1010	69	4 ½	50	55	22.0	130	1450	6
Sides										
corn	4 oz.	120	21	1 ½	3	0	0.0	0	45	3
French fries, salted	1 (5 oz.)	430	50	3	5	23	5.0	0	95	5
garlic bread	2 pieces	170	21	4	9	2.0	0	350	1	
mashed potatoes	4 oz.	100	55	3 ½	2	3	2.0	5	350	1
onion rings	1 (5 oz.)	520	48	3	6	36	2.0	0	980	3
red-skinned potatoes	4 oz.	210	27	2	4	7	2.0	0	630	3
sauteed spinach	2 oz.	70	5	0	1	6	1.0	0	125	2
seasoned fries	1 (5 oz.)	630	48	3	6	47	9.0	0	1010	5
vegetable rice pilaf	5 oz.	190	35	2	4	3	0.0	0	490	2
Domino's Pizza®										
BBQ Buffalo wings	2	230	6	½	17	14	3.5	50	410	0
Breadsticks	1	110	11	1	2	6	1.5	0	100	0
Brooklyn style pizza, large, (14 in.)										
w/ pepperoni	1/6 pie	300	27	2	14	16	6.5	40	810	1
w/ sausage	1/6 pie	330	29	2	15	18	7.5	45	830	1
Cheese pizza, medium, (12 in.)										
deep dish	1/8 pie	260	29	2	10	12	5.0	25	630	3
hand tossed	1/8 pie	210	25	1 ½	8	8	3.5	20	460	1
thin crust	¼ pie	330	30	2	14	18	7.0	40	660	3
Cheesy bread	1 piece	120	11	1	4	6	2.0	5	140	0
Chocolate lava crunch cake	1 cake	350	47	3	4	17	10.0	65	170	1
Deluxe Feast®	1/8 pie	230	27	2	9	10	4.0	20	550	2
Extra cheese pizza, medium, (12 in.)										
deep dish	1/8 pie	290	30	2	12	14	7.0	35	740	3
hand tossed	1/8 pie	230	26	2	10	10	5.0	25	540	1
thin crust	¼ pie	380	31	2	16	21	10.0	50	810	3
Ham pizza, medium, (12 in.)										
deep dish	1/8 pie	240	28	2	10	10	4.0	20	655	3
hand tossed	1/8 pie	195	25	1 ½	8	7	2.5	20	515	1
thin crust	¼ pie	305	29	2	14	15	5.5	35	750	2
Hot Buffalo wings	2	200	2	0	16	14	3.5	50	690	0

FAST FOODS & RESTAURANT CHAINS
Domino's Pizza®

ITEM	AMOUNT	CALORIES	CARBOHYDRATE (g)	CARBOHYDRATE CHOICES	PROTEIN (g)	FAT (g)	SATURATED FAT (g)	CHOLESTEROL (mg)	SODIUM (mg)	FIBER (g)
Pepperoni pizza, medium, (12 in.)										
deep dish	1/8 pie	260	28	2	10	12	5.0	20	660	3
hand tossed	1/8 pie	210	25	1 ½	8	9	3.5	20	450	1
thin crust	¼ pie	340	29	2	14	19	7.5	40	760	2
Sausage pizza, medium, (12 in.)										
deep dish	1/8 pie	275	29	2	11	13	5.5	20	660	3
hand tossed	1/8 pie	230	26	2	9	10	4.0	20	520	1
thin crust	¼ pie	370	30	2	14	21	8.5	40	760	2

Dunkin' Donuts®

ITEM	AMOUNT	CALORIES	CARBOHYDRATE (g)	CARBOHYDRATE CHOICES	PROTEIN (g)	FAT (g)	SATURATED FAT (g)	CHOLESTEROL (mg)	SODIUM (mg)	FIBER (g)
Bagel twists										
cheddar cheese	1	400	63	4	17	9	4.5	20	800	5
cinnamon raisin	1	350	72	4 ½	11	4	0.5	0	460	5
French toast	1	330	66	4 ½	10	3	0.0	0	540	4
Bagels										
blueberry	1	330	65	4	11	3	1.0	0	620	5
cinnamon raisin	1	330	65	4	11	4	0.5	0	450	5
everything	1	350	66	4	13	5	0.5	0	660	5
garlic	1	340	68	4	12	3	0.5	0	660	6
multigrain	1	390	65	4	14	8	0.5	0	560	9
onion	1	310	63	4	11	2	0.0	0	380	3
plain	1	320	63	4	11	3	0.5	0	660	5
poppy seed	1	350	64	4	13	6	0.5	0	660	5
salt	1	320	63	4	11	3	0.5	0	3420	5
sesame	1	360	63	4	13	6	0.5	0	660	5
wheat	1	320	61	4	12	4	0.0	0	550	5
Breakfast sandwiches										
bagel, w/ egg & cheese	1	480	66	4	20	15	5.0	200	1130	5
bagel, w/ sausage egg & cheese	1	680	67	4	29	32	12.0	250	1590	5
biscuit, w/ egg & cheese	1	440	35	2	14	27	13.0	200	1090	1
croissant, w/ egg & cheese	1	480	38	2 ½	16	29	12.0	200	820	2
croissant, w/ ham, egg & cheese	1	510	38	2 ½	21	31	12.0	215	1080	2
egg white & cheese Wake-Up Wrap®	1	150	13	1	8	7	3.0	10	480	1
egg white turkey sausage flatbread	1	290	34	2	21	8	3.0	20	600	3
egg white veggie flatbread	1	330	35	2	20	12	5.0	25	820	4
English muffin, w/ bacon, egg & cheese	1	370	34	2	18	18	6.0	205	1030	1
English muffin, w/ egg & cheese	1	320	34	2	14	15	5.0	200	820	1
English muffin, w/ egg white & cheese	1	250	33	2	15	7	3.0	10	830	1
Coffee										
black	small	5	1	0	0	0	0.0	0	5	0
black	medium	10	1	0	1	0	0.0	0	10	0
black	large	10	2	0	1	0	0.0	0	15	0

FAST FOODS & RESTAURANT CHAINS
Dunkin' Donuts®

ITEM	AMOUNT	CALORIES	CARBOHYDRATE (g)	CARBOHYDRATE CHOICES	PROTEIN (g)	FAT (g)	SATURATED FAT (g)	CHOLESTEROL (mg)	SODIUM (mg)	FIBER (g)
Coffee *(continued)*										
flavored, black, most varieties	small	10	1	0	0	0	0.0	0	5	0
w/ cream & sugar	small	120	19	1	1	6	4.0	20	20	0
w/ cream, w/o sugar	small	60	2	0	1	6	4.0	20	20	0
w/ milk & sugar	small	80	20	1	1	1	1.0	5	20	0
w/ skim milk & sugar	small	70	20	1	2	0	0.0	0	25	0
w/ skim milk, w/o sugar	small	15	3	0	2	0	0.0	0	25	0
Cookies										
oatmeal raisin	1	320	54	3 ½	5	9	4.5	30	210	3
reverse chocolate chunk	1	380	50	3	5	18	10.0	40	320	2
triple chocolate chunk	1	360	53	3 ½	5	15	8.0	35	380	2
Coolattas®										
coffee w/ cream	small	400	49	3	3	23	14.0	80	75	0
coffee w/ milk	small	240	50	3	4	4	2.5	15	90	0
coffee w/ skim milk	small	210	51	3 ½	4	0	0.0	0	90	0
strawberry fruit	small	310	75	5	0	0	0.0	0	45	0
Tropicana® orange	small	230	57	4	1	0	0.0	0	40	0
vanilla bean	small	430	91	6	3	6	3.5	20	170	0
Cream cheese										
plain	1	150	3	0	3	15	9.0	40	250	0
plain, reduced fat	1	100	5	0	4	8	5.0	25	250	0
strawberry, reduced fat	1	150	15	1	2	10	6.0	30	200	0
veggie, reduced fat	1	120	6	½	2	10	6.0	30	240	0
Danish										
apple cheese	1	330	41	3	4	16	7.0	0	270	1
cheese	1	330	39	2 ½	5	17	8.0	5	270	1
strawberry	1	320	40	2 ½	4	16	7.0	0	260	1
Donuts										
Bavarian kreme	1	270	31	2	4	15	7.0	0	350	1
blueberry cake	1	340	44	3	4	17	8.0	30	570	1
Boston kreme	1	310	39	2 ½	3	16	7.0	0	370	1
bow tie	1	310	39	2 ½	4	15	7.0	0	400	1
chocolate frosted	1	270	31	2	3	15	7.0	0	340	1
chocolate frosted cake	1	370	45	3	4	23	10.0	25	320	1
chocolate glazed cake	1	370	35	2	3	24	11.0	0	390	1
coffee roll	1	400	53	3 ½	7	18	7.0	0	400	3
eclair	1	390	52	3 ½	5	19	8.0	0	360	2
French cruller	1	250	18	1	2	20	9.0	35	105	0
gingerbread	1	310	42	3	4	14	6.0	25	360	1
glazed	1	260	31	2	3	14	6.0	0	330	1
glazed cake stick	1	370	48	3	4	18	8.0	35	420	1
jelly filled	1	290	36	2 ½	3	14	7.0	0	340	1

FAST FOODS & RESTAURANT CHAINS
Dunkin' Donuts®

ITEM	AMOUNT	CALORIES	CARBOHYDRATE (g)	CARBOHYDRATE CHOICES	PROTEIN (g)	FAT (g)	SATURATED FAT (g)	CHOLESTEROL (mg)	SODIUM (mg)	FIBER (g)
Donuts *(continued)*										
jelly stick	1	420	60	4	4	18	8.0	35	440	1
strawberry frosted	1	280	32	2	3	15	7.0	0	340	1
vanilla kreme filled	1	380	42	3	4	23	10.0	0	370	1
Dunkaccino®	small	240	35	2	2	11	9.0	10	220	1
Hot chocolate	small	220	39	2 ½	2	7	7.0	0	270	2
Hot espresso drinks										
cappuccino	small	80	7	½	4	4	2.5	15	70	0
cappuccino w/sugar	small	140	24	1 ½	4	4	2.5	15	70	0
espresso	1 shot	5	1	0	0	0	0.0	0	5	0
gingerbread latte	small	220	34	2	8	6	3.5	25	140	0
latte	small	120	10	½	6	6	3.5	25	105	0
latte, lite	small	80	13	1	7	0	0.0	0	110	0
pumpkin latte	small	210	32	2	8	6	4.0	25	140	0
vanilla latte lite	small	90	14	1	7	0	0.0	0	110	0
Iced coffees										
black	small	10	2	0	1	0	0.0	0	5	0
black	medium	15	2	0	1	0	0.0	0	10	0
black	large	20	3	0	1	0	0.0	0	15	0
black, w/ sugar	small	70	19	1	1	0	0.0	0	5	0
w/ cream & sugar	small	120	20	1	1	6	4.0	20	20	3
w/ cream, no sugar	small	70	3	0	1	6	4.0	20	20	0
w/ milk & sugar	small	90	21	1 ½	2	1	1.0	5	20	0
w/ milk, no sugar	small	30	3	0	2	1	1.0	5	20	0
w/ skim milk & sugar	small	80	21	1 ½	2	0	0.0	0	25	0
w/ skim milk, no sugar	small	20	3	0	2	0	0.0	0	25	0
Muffins										
blueberry	1	480	81	5 ½	6	15	1.5	15	470	2
blueberry, reduced fat	1	430	80	5	6	9	1.0	15	650	2
chocolate chip	1	590	92	6	7	22	6.0	20	490	3
coffee cake	1	630	95	6	7	25	7.0	15	510	1
corn	1	490	80	5	6	16	1.5	20	820	1
gingerbread	1	530	82	5 ½	9	19	3.5	75	660	2
honey raisin bran	1	480	82	5	6	13	1.5	15	430	5
pumpkin	1	600	83	5 ½	7	26	6.0	55	520	3
Munchkins										
cinnamon cake	1	60	6	½	1	4	1.5	5	65	0
glazed	1	70	7	½	1	4	2.0	0	80	0
glazed cake	1	70	8	½	1	4	1.5	5	65	0
glazed chocolate cake	1	70	8	½	1	4	1.5	0	85	0
jelly filled	1	80	9	½	1	4	2.0	0	85	0
plain cake	1	60	6	½	1	4	1.5	5	65	0

Dunkin' Donuts®

ITEM	AMOUNT	CALORIES	CARBOHYDRATE (g)	CARBOHYDRATE CHOICES	PROTEIN (g)	FAT (g)	SATURATED FAT (g)	CHOLESTEROL (mg)	SODIUM (mg)	FIBER (g)
Munchkins *(continued)*										
powdered cake	1	60	7	½	1	4	1.5	5	65	0
sugared	1	60	6	½	1	4	1.5	5	65	0
Turbo shot	small	5	1	0	0	0	0.0	0	5	0
Vanilla chai tea	medium	330	53	3 ½	11	8	8.0	10	180	1

Hardee's®

ITEM	AMOUNT	CALORIES	CARBOHYDRATE (g)	CARBOHYDRATE CHOICES	PROTEIN (g)	FAT (g)	SATURATED FAT (g)	CHOLESTEROL (mg)	SODIUM (mg)	FIBER (g)
Apple turnover, w/o topping	1	270	35	2	3	13	3.5	5	260	1
Biscuits										
bacon, w/ egg & cheese	1	530	36	2 ½	15	36	11.0	195	1390	0
Biscuit 'N' Gravy™	1	530	47	3	8	34	8.0	10	1550	0
chicken fillet	1	620	47	3	24	37	8.0	50	1560	1
Cinnamon 'N' Raisin™	1	300	40	2 ½	3	15	3.0	0	680	1
country ham	1	440	36	2 ½	14	26	6.0	35	1710	0
Monster Biscuit™	1	770	37	2 ½	29	55	18.0	250	2310	0
smoked sausage	1	620	37	2 ½	14	46	n/a	n/a	1680	0
Chicken sandwiches										
big chicken fillet	1	710	62	4	33	38	7.0	55	1610	5
charbroiled BBQ	1	400	62	4	27	6	1.0	45	1370	5
Fish supreme sandwich	1	630	51	3 ½	22	38	7.0	40	1310	3
French fries, natural-cut										
small	1 order	320	45	3	4	14	3.0	0	710	4
medium	1 order	430	60	4	5	19	4.0	5	960	4
large	1 order	470	65	4	5	21	4.0	5	1640	4
Frisco Breakfast Sandwich®	1	420	39	2 ½	25	18	7.0	215	1250	2
Grits	1 order	110	16	1	2	5	n/a	n/a	480	0
Hamburgers										
cheeseburger, regular	1	350	32	2	16	19	n/a	n/a	730	1
hamburger, regular	1	310	32	2	14	15	4.0	35	500	1
⅓ lb. Bacon Cheese Thickburger®	1	850	49	3	38	57	19.0	105	1650	3
⅓ lb. Cheeseburger Thickburger®	1	620	51	3 ½	35	33	13.0	80	1580	3
⅓ lb. Frisco Thickburger®	1	930	42	3	44	64	21.0	125	1840	2
⅓ lb. Original Thickburger®	1	860	52	3 ½	35	58	17.0	105	1630	4
⅔ lb. Monster Thickburger®	1	1320	46	3	70	95	n/a	n/a	3020	2
Hot Ham 'N' Cheese™ sandwich	1	460	40	2 ½	36	20	n/a	n/a	2040	2
Jumbo chili dog	1	400	25	1 ½	16	26	9.0	55	1170	1
Turkey burger	1	460	47	3	31	17	n/a	n/a	930	4

KFC®

ITEM	AMOUNT	CALORIES	CARBOHYDRATE (g)	CARBOHYDRATE CHOICES	PROTEIN (g)	FAT (g)	SATURATED FAT (g)	CHOLESTEROL (mg)	SODIUM (mg)	FIBER (g)
BBQ baked beans	1 order	210	41	2 ½	8	2	0.0	0	780	8
Biscuit	1	180	23	1 ½	4	8	6.0	0	530	1

FAST FOODS & RESTAURANT CHAINS

KFC

ITEM	AMOUNT	CALORIES	CARBOHYDRATE (g)	CARBOHYDRATE CHOICES	PROTEIN (g)	FAT (g)	SATURATED FAT (g)	CHOLESTEROL (mg)	SODIUM (mg)	FIBER (g)
Chicken sandwiches										
doublicious grilled filet, w/o sauce	1	340	32	2	35	8	3.5	80	880	2
honey BBQ flavored	1	320	47	3	24	4	1.0	70	770	3
Chunky chicken pot pie	1	790	66	4 ½	29	45	37.0	75	1970	3
Cole slaw	1 order	180	20	1	1	10	1.5	5	150	2
Colonel's Crispy Strips®	3 pieces	340	27	2	33	11	4.0	70	1280	3
Corn on the cob	1 (3 inch)	70	16	1	2	1	0.0	0	0	2
Extra Crispy® chicken										
breast	1	510	16	1	39	33	7.0	110	1010	0
drumstick	1	150	5	0	12	10	2.0	55	360	0
thigh	1	340	10	½	20	24	5.0	80	780	0
whole wing	1	190	6	½	12	13	2.5	55	410	0
Fiery Buffalo Hot Wings®	1	70	5	0	4	4	0.5	20	270	0
Green beans	1 order	20	3	0	1	0	0.0	0	290	1
Hot Wings®	1 piece	70	4	0	4	4	0.5	20	140	0
KFC® Famous Bowl™, w/ mashed potato & gravy	1 order	680	74	5	26	31	8.0	45	2130	6
Macaroni & cheese	1 order	160	19	1	5	7	2.5	5	720	1
Mashed potatoes, w/ gravy	1 order	120	19	1	2	4	1.0	0	530	1
Original Recipe® chicken										
breast	1	360	11	1	34	21	5.0	110	1080	0
breast, w/o skin or breading	1	160	2	0	31	4	1.0	85	580	0
drumstick	1	120	3	0	11	7	1.5	45	310	0
thigh	1	250	7	½	17	17	4.5	80	730	0
whole wing	1	120	3	0	11	7	1.5	50	380	0
Popcorn chicken										
kids	1 order	260	12	1	15	17	3.5	30	690	1
individual	1 order	400	18	1	22	26	6.0	45	1040	1
large	1 order	560	26	2	32	37	8.0	65	1480	2
Potato salad	1 order	210	26	2	2	11	2.5	10	560	3
Potato wedges	1 order	310	32	2	4	18	3.0	0	870	4

McDonald's®

ITEM	AMOUNT	CALORIES	CARBOHYDRATE (g)	CARBOHYDRATE CHOICES	PROTEIN (g)	FAT (g)	SATURATED FAT (g)	CHOLESTEROL (mg)	SODIUM (mg)	FIBER (g)
Biscuits, regular size										
bacon, egg & cheese	1	420	37	2 ½	15	23	12.0	235	1160	2
sausage	1	430	34	2	11	27	12.0	30	1080	2
sausage & egg	1	510	36	2 ½	18	33	14.0	250	1170	2
Chicken McNuggets®	4 pieces	190	11	1	10	12	2.0	30	400	0
Chicken sandwiches										
classic, grilled	1	420	51	3 ½	32	10	2.0	70	1190	3
crispy chicken classic	1	530	59	4	28	20	3.5	50	1150	3

FAST FOODS & RESTAURANT CHAINS
McDonald's®

ITEM	AMOUNT	CALORIES	CARBOHYDRATE (g)	CARBOHYDRATE CHOICES	PROTEIN (g)	FAT (g)	SATURATED FAT (g)	CHOLESTEROL (mg)	SODIUM (mg)	FIBER (g)
Chicken sandwiches *(continued)*										
Honey Mustard Snack Wrap™										
w/ crispy chicken	1	330	34	2	14	16	4.5	30	780	1
w/ grilled chicken	1	260	27	2	18	9	3.5	45	800	1
McChicken®	1	360	40	2 ½	14	16	3.0	35	830	2
Chicken Selects®	3 pieces	400	23	1 ½	23	24	3.5	50	1010	0
Cinnamon melts	1 order	460	66	4 ½	6	19	9.0	15	370	3
Egg McMuffin®	1	300	30	2	18	12	5.0	260	820	2
Filet-O-Fish®	1	380	38	2 ½	15	18	3.5	40	640	2
French fries	medium	380	48	3	4	19	2.5	0	270	5
Fruit 'n yogurt parfait	1 (7oz.)	160	31	2	4	2	1.0	5	85	1
Hamburgers										
Big Mac®	1	540	45	3	25	29	10.0	75	1040	3
Big N' Tasty®	1	460	37	2 ½	24	24	8.0	70	720	3
Big N' Tasty®, w/ cheese	1	510	38	2 ½	27	28	11.0	85	960	3
cheeseburger	1	300	33	2	15	12	6.0	40	750	2
double cheeseburger	1	440	34	2	25	23	11.0	80	1150	2
hamburger	1	250	31	2	12	9	3.5	25	520	2
Quarter Pounder®, w/ cheese	1	510	40	2 ½	29	26	12.0	90	1190	3
Hash browns	1	150	15	1	1	9	1.5	0	310	2
Hot cakes, w/o marg. & syrup	1 order	350	60	4	8	9	2.0	20	590	3
Ice cream cone, vanilla, reduced fat	1	150	24	1 ½	4	3.5	2.0	15	60	0
McFlurry®										
M&M®	1 (12.5 oz.)	710	105	7	15	25	16.0	60	220	4
Oreo®	1 (11.6 oz.)	580	89	6	13	19	10.0	50	320	3
McGriddle®										
bacon, egg & cheese	1	420	48	3	15	18	8.0	240	1110	2
sausage	1	420	44	3	11	22	8.0	35	1030	2
sausage, egg & cheese	1	560	48	3	20	32	12.0	265	1360	2
McSkillet™, w/ sausage	1	610	44	3	27	36	14.0	410	1390	3
Salad dressings, Newman's Own®										
balsamic, low fat	1 pkt.	40	4	0	0	3	0.0	0	730	0
creamy Caesar	1 pkt.	190	4	0	2	18	3.5	20	500	0
creamy Southwest	1 pkt.	100	11	1	1	6	1.0	20	340	0
Italian, low fat	1 pkt.	60	8	½	1	3	0.0	0	730	0
ranch	1 pkt.	170	9	½	1	15	2.5	20	530	0
Salads										
bacon ranch, w/ crispy chicken	1	370	20	1	29	20	6.0	75	970	3
bacon ranch, w/ grilled chicken	1	260	12	1	33	9	4.0	90	1010	3
bacon ranch, w/o chicken	1	140	10	½	9	7	3.5	25	300	3
Caesar, w/ crispy chicken	1	1330	20	1	26	17	4.5	60	840	3
Caesar, w/ grilled chicken	1	1220	12	1	30	6	3.0	75	890	3

FAST FOODS & RESTAURANT CHAINS

McDonald's®

ITEM	AMOUNT	CALORIES	CARBOHYDRATE (g)	CARBOHYDRATE CHOICES	PROTEIN (g)	FAT (g)	SATURATED FAT (g)	CHOLESTEROL (mg)	SODIUM (mg)	FIBER (g)
Salads *(continued)*										
Caesar, w/o chicken	1	190	9	½	7	4	2.5	10	180	3
garden, side salad	1	120	4	0	1	0	0.0	0	10	1
Southwest, w/ crispy chicken	1	1430	38	2	26	20	4.0	55	920	6
Southwest, w/ grilled chicken	1	1320	30	2	30	9	3.0	70	960	6
Southwest, w/o chicken	1	1140	20	1	6	5	2.0	10	150	6
Sausage McMuffin®, w/ egg	1	450	30	2	21	27	10.0	285	920	2
Shakes, Triple Thick®										
chocolate	1 (16 fl. oz.)	580	102	7	13	14	8.0	50	250	1
strawberry	1 (16 fl. oz.)	560	97	6 ½	13	13	8.0	50	170	0
vanilla	1 (16 fl. oz.)	550	96	6 ½	13	13	8.0	50	190	0
Sundaes										
hot caramel	1	1340	60	4	7	8	5.0	30	160	1
hot fudge	1	330	54	3 ½	8	10	7.0	25	180	2
strawberry	1	1280	49	3	6	6	4.0	25	95	1
Value meals, regular, w/ medium drink & medium fries										
Big Mac®	1 meal	1130	151	10	29	48	12.5	75	1325	8
Chicken Selects®, 3 piece	1 meal	990	129	8 ½	27	43	6.0	50	1295	5
double cheeseburger	1 meal	1030	140	9	29	42	13.5	80	1435	7
Filet-O-Fish®	1 meal	970	144	9	19	37	6.0	40	925	7
Quarter Pounder®	1 meal	1000	143	9	28	38	9.5	65	1015	7

Olive Garden®

Garden Fare® Selections

ITEM	AMOUNT	CALORIES	CARBOHYDRATE (g)	CARBOHYDRATE CHOICES	PROTEIN (g)	FAT (g)	SATURATED FAT (g)	CHOLESTEROL (mg)	SODIUM (mg)	FIBER (g)
Appetizers										
breadstick, w/ garlic-butter spread	1 order	150	28	2	n/a	2	0.0	n/a	400	2
bruschetta	1 order	610	100	6	n/a	13	2.5	n/a	1760	10
calamari, w/ marinara sauce	1 order	960	74	5	n/a	57	5.0	n/a	2880	5
calamari, w/o sauce	1 order	890	64	4	n/a	54	5.0	n/a	2340	2
Caprese flatbread	1 order	600	46	3	n/a	36	11.0	n/a	1520	5
mussels di Napoli	1 order	180	13	1	n/a	8	4.0	n/a	1770	0
stuffed mushrooms	1 order	280	15	1	n/a	19	5.0	n/a	720	3
Chicken dishes, dinner portions, as served										
chicken Alfredo	1 order	1440	103	6 ½	n/a	82	48.0	n/a	2070	5
chicken Marsala	1 order	770	59	3 ½	n/a	37	5.0	n/a	1800	16
chicken parmigiana	1 order	1090	79	4	n/a	49	18.0	n/a	3380	27
chicken scampi	1 order	1070	88	5 ½	n/a	53	20.0	n/a	2220	8
garlic-herb chicken con broccoli	1 order	960	90	5 ½	n/a	41	18.0	n/a	2180	12
stuffed chicken Marsala	1 order	800	40	2 ½	n/a	36	16.0	n/a	2830	6
Venetian apricot chicken	1 order	380	32	2	n/a	4	1.5	n/a	1420	8
Desserts										
black tie mousse cake	1 order	760	73	4 ½	n/a	48	27.0	n/a	270	8

FAST FOODS & RESTAURANT CHAINS
Olive Garden®

ITEM	AMOUNT	CALORIES	CARBOHYDRATE (g)	CARBOHYDRATE CHOICES	PROTEIN (g)	FAT (g)	SATURATED FAT (g)	CHOLESTEROL (mg)	SODIUM (mg)	FIBER (g)
Desserts (continued)										
dolcini, chocolate mousse	1 order	290	23	1 ½	n/a	21	10.0	n/a	120	2
dolcini, limoncello mousse	1 order	230	28	2	n/a	13	8.0	n/a	70	0
dolcini, strawberry & white chocolate	1 order	210	27	2	n/a	11	6.0	n/a	70	0
tiramisu	1 order	510	48	3	n/a	32	19.0	n/a	75	2
warm apple crostata	1 order	730	104	7	n/a	32	15.0	n/a	240	6
white chocolate raspberry cheesecake	1 order	890	70	4 ½	n/a	62	36.0	n/a	490	6
Pasta dishes, dinner portions, as served										
capellini pomodoro	1 order	840	141	9	n/a	17	3.0	n/a	1250	19
cheese ravioli, w/ meat sauce	1 order	790	88	5 ½	n/a	28	14.0	n/a	1510	12
eggplant parmigiana	1 order	850	98	6	n/a	35	10.0	n/a	1900	19
fettuccine Alfredo	1 order	1220	99	6 ½	n/a	75	47.0	n/a	1350	5
five cheese ziti al forno	1 order	1050	112	7	n/a	48	26.0	n/a	2370	9
lasagna classico	1 order	850	39	2	n/a	47	25.0	n/a	2830	19
spaghetti & meatballs	1 order	1110	103	6 ½	n/a	50	20.0	n/a	2180	9
spaghetti, w/ meat sauce	1 order	710	94	6	n/a	22	8.0	n/a	1340	9
tour of Italy	1 order	1450	97	6	n/a	74	33.0	n/a	3830	10
Salads										
garden-fresh, w/ dressing	1 serving	350	22	1 ½	n/a	26	4.5	n/a	1930	3
garden-fresh, w/o dressing	1 serving	120	17	1	n/a	3.5	0.5	n/a	550	3
Seafood dishes, dinner portions, as served										
capellini di mare	1 order	650	82	5	n/a	18	5.0	n/a	1830	7
grilled shrimp Caprese	1 order	990	83	5	n/a	54	28.0	n/a	2990	7
seafood Alfredo	1 order	1020	88	5 ½	n/a	52	31.0	n/a	2430	9
shrimp primavera	1 order	730	110	7	n/a	12	2.0	n/a	1620	14
Soups										
minestrone	1 order	100	18	1	n/a	1	0.0	n/a	1020	3
pasta e fagioli	1 order	130	17	1	n/a	3	1.0	n/a	680	6
zuppa Toscana	1 order	170	24	1 ½	n/a	4	2.0	n/a	960	2

P.F. Chang's China Bistro®
Appetizers

ITEM	AMOUNT	CALORIES	CARBOHYDRATE (g)	CARBOHYDRATE CHOICES	PROTEIN (g)	FAT (g)	SATURATED FAT (g)	CHOLESTEROL (mg)	SODIUM (mg)	FIBER (g)
Chang's chicken lettuce wrap (Servings per dish = ~4)	1 serving	160	17	1	8	7	1.0	n/a	650	2
Chang's vegetarian lettuce wraps (Servings per dish = ~3½)	1 serving	140	11	1	6	7	1.0	n/a	530	2
Crab wontons, w/o sauce (Servings per dish = ~3)	1 serving	163	13	1	5	10	4.0	n/a	303	0
Egg rolls (Servings per dish = ~2)	1 serving	174	22	1 ½	5	8	1.0	n/a	673	3

FAST FOODS & RESTAURANT CHAINS

P.F. Chang's China Bistro® – Appetizers

ITEM	AMOUNT	CALORIES	CARBOHYDRATE (g)	CARBOHYDRATE CHOICES	PROTEIN (g)	FAT (g)	SATURATED FAT (g)	CHOLESTEROL (mg)	SODIUM (mg)	FIBER (g)
Pork dumplings, steamed (Servings per dish = ~6)	1 serving	60	6	½	4	2	1.0	n/a	125	0
Salt & pepper calamari (Servings per dish = ~4)	1 serving	160	11	1	6	10	2.0	n/a	208	0
Seared Ahi tuna (Servings per dish = ~2)	1 serving	160	7	½	10	11	2.0	n/a	860	1
Shanghai cucumbers (Servings per dish = ~1½)	1 serving	40	3	0	2	2	0.0	n/a	743	1
Shrimp dumplings, pan fried (Servings per dish = ~6)	1 serving	60	6	½	4	2	0.0	n/a	170	0
Vegetable dumplings (Servings per dish = ~6)	1 serving	45	8	½	2	0	0.0	n/a	80	0
Entrées										
Almond & cashew chicken (Servings per dish = ~3)	1 serving	373	24	1 ½	29	18	3.0	n/a	1960	2
Beef à la Szechuan (Servings per dish = ~3)	1 serving	303	25	1 ½	22	12	3.0	n/a	1084	1
Beef w/ broccoli (Servings per dish = ~3)	1 serving	290	21	1 ½	24	12	3.0	n/a	1573	2
Buddha's feast, steamed (Servings per dish = ~2)	1 serving	55	11	1	4	0	0.0	n/a	40	4
Buddha's feast, stir-fried (Servings per dish = ~2)	1 serving	220	29	2	14	6	1.0	n/a	1620	5
Cantonese scallops (Servings per dish = ~2)	1 serving	245	17	1	15	14	2.0	n/a	1000	2
Cantonese shrimp (Servings per dish = ~2)	1 serving	215	10	½	21	10	2.0	n/a	950	2
Chang's lemon scallops (Servings per dish = ~3)	1 serving	243	28	2	11	10	2.0	n/a	540	1
Chang's spicy chicken (Servings per dish = ~3)	1 serving	323	23	1 ½	28	13	2.0	n/a	550	0
Chicken w/ black bean sauce (Servings per dish = ~3)	1 serving	300	14	1	29	16	2.0	n/a	1850	0
Coconut curry vegetables (Servings per dish = ~2)	1 serving	510	26	1 ½	22	36	12.0	n/a	650	5
Combo double pan fried noodles (Servings per dish = ~4)	1 serving	455	44	3	16	21	2.0	n/a	1923	1
Crispy honey chicken (Servings per dish = ~3)	1 serving	477	49	3	16	23	4.0	n/a	510	0
Crispy honey shrimp (Servings per dish = ~2)	1 serving	460	55	3 ½	10	22	4.0	n/a	805	1

FAST FOODS & RESTAURANT CHAINS

P.F. Chang's China Bistro® – Entrées

ITEM	AMOUNT	CALORIES	CARBOHYDRATE (g)	CARBOHYDRATE CHOICES	PROTEIN (g)	FAT (g)	SATURATED FAT (g)	CHOLESTEROL (mg)	SODIUM (mg)	FIBER (g)
Dan-Dan noodles (Servings per dish = ~4)	1 serving	270	30	2	13	7	1.0	n/a	1388	2
Garlic noodles (Servings per dish = ~4)	1 serving	178	31	2	5	4	1.0	n/a	360	1
Garlic snap peas, small (Servings per dish = ~1½)	1 serving	64	7	½	2	2	0.0	n/a	107	2
Ginger chicken & broccoli (Servings per dish = ~3)	1 serving	273	18	1	28	11	2.0	n/a	1457	2
Hot fish, Hunan style (Servings per dish = ~3)	1 serving	340	21	1 ½	16	22	3.0	n/a	1043	1
Kung pao chicken (Servings per dish = ~3)	1 serving	383	14	1	33	23	4.0	n/a	940	2
Lemon pepper shrimp (Servings per dish = ~2)	1 serving	235	19	1	21	10	2.0	n/a	1080	3
Ma po tofu (Servings per dish = ~3)	1 serving	350	17	1	20	23	5.0	n/a	1060	2
Mongolian beef (Servings per dish = ~3)	1 serving	337	20	1	29	15	4.0	n/a	1340	1
Moo goo gai pan (Servings per dish = ~3)	1 serving	247	13	1	18	13	2.0	n/a	823	1
Mu shu chicken (Servings per dish = ~2)	1 serving	285	16	1	26	13	3.0	n/a	1540	3
Mu shu pork (Servings per dish = ~2)	1 serving	320	16	1	21	19	7.0	n/a	2275	3
Oolong marinated sea bass (Servings per dish = ~2)	1 serving	315	15	1	24	19	5.0	n/a	1550	2
Orange peel beef (Servings per dish = ~3)	1 serving	283	21	1 ½	12	13	3.0	n/a	833	1
Orange peel chicken (Servings per dish = ~3)	1 serving	333	20	1	29	15	3.0	n/a	770	1
Orange peel shrimp (Servings per dish = ~3)	1 serving	187	14	1	15	14	1.0	n/a	937	1
P.F. Chang's® fried rice combo (Servings per dish = ~4)	1 serving	363	41	3	19	13	3.0	n/a	1063	1
Singapore street noodles (Servings per dish = ~3)	1 serving	300	42	3	11	6	1.0	n/a	1157	3
Spinach w/ garlic, small (Servings per dish = ~1½)	1 serving	53	5	0	4	3	1.0	n/a	300	3
Stir-fried eggplant (Servings per dish = ~4)	1 serving	270	14	1	2	22	3.0	n/a	760	2
Sweet & sour pork (Servings per dish = ~2)	1 serving	460	72	5	14	14	7.0	n/a	950	2

FAST FOODS & RESTAURANT CHAINS

P.F. Chang's China Bistro® – Entrées

ITEM	AMOUNT	CALORIES	CARBOHYDRATE (g)	CARBOHYDRATE CHOICES	PROTEIN (g)	FAT (g)	SATURATED FAT (g)	CHOLESTEROL (mg)	SODIUM (mg)	FIBER (g)
Szechwan asparagus, small (Servings per dish = ~1½)	1 serving	100	10	½	3	6	1.0	n/a	730	2
Soups & salads										
Chicken chopped salad, w/ ginger dressing (Servings per dish = ~2)	1 serving	365	13	1	23	24	4.0	n/a	640	2
Hot & sour soup (Servings per dish = ~5)	1 serving	80	9	½	5	3	1.0	n/a	1000	0
Wonton soup (Servings per dish = ~5)	1 serving	92	9	½	7	3	1.0	n/a	482	0
Panera Bread®										
Bagels										
asiago	1	330	55	3 ½	13	6	3.5	10	580	2
blueberry	1	330	68	4 ½	10	2	0.0	0	490	2
cinnamon crunch	1	430	80	5	9	8	5.0	0	430	2
everything	1	300	59	4	10	3	0.0	0	640	2
plain	1	290	59	4	10	2	0.0	0	460	2
whole grain	1	340	67	4	13	3	0.0	0	400	6
Breads										
French baguette side	1 (2.5 oz.)	180	36	2 ½	6	1	0.0	0	440	1
whole grain baguette side	1 (2.5 oz.)	180	36	2 ½	7	2	0.0	0	400	4
Breakfast sandwiches										
bacon, egg & cheese on asiago bagel	1	610	55	3 ½	33	27	13.0	225	1250	2
grilled egg & cheese on ciabatta	1	380	43	3	18	14	6.0	190	620	2
power	1	330	31	2	22	14	6.0	200	830	4
sausage, egg & cheese on French toast bagel	1	540	44	3	26	28	11.0	230	950	2
Egg soufflés										
four cheese	1	480	36	2 ½	16	29	16.0	195	700	2
ham & Swiss	1	490	35	2	19	30	16.0	175	760	2
spinach artichoke	1	540	38	2 ½	20	34	19.0	165	910	2
Hot Paninis										
Cuban chicken	1	860	86	6	46	36	10.0	100	1770	4
Fontega Chicken®	1	850	79	5	49	38	9.0	110	1910	4
smokehouse turkey	1	690	64	4	52	25	12.0	100	2350	4
tomato mozzarella	1	770	96	6	30	29	10.0	35	1290	6
turkey artichoke	1	740	86	5 ½	41	26	8.0	50	2200	5
Pastries & sweets										
apple pastry	1	380	44	3	7	17	13.0	20	320	1
artisan chocolate pastry	1	410	46	3	8	22	14.0	50	260	2
bear claw	1	550	67	4 ½	10	28	12.0	65	360	3

FAST FOODS & RESTAURANT CHAINS
Panera Bread®

ITEM	AMOUNT	CALORIES	CARBOHYDRATE (g)	CARBOHYDRATE CHOICES	PROTEIN (g)	FAT (g)	SATURATED FAT (g)	CHOLESTEROL (mg)	SODIUM (mg)	FIBER (g)
Pastries & sweets *(continued)*										
carrot walnut muffin	1	500	72	5	8	21	4.5	65	580	3
chocolate chip muffie	1	320	46	3	4	14	4.0	40	200	2
chocolate chipper cookie	1	440	59	4	5	23	14.0	60	250	2
chocolate fudge brownie	1	410	64	4	5	14	8.0	85	260	2
cinnamon crumb coffee cake	1	470	54	3 ½	6	25	9.0	105	310	1
cornbread muffie	1	230	33	2	3	9	1.5	35	250	1
French croissant	1	310	30	2	7	18	11.0	60	260	1
orange scone	1	470	87	6	4	11	7.0	45	460	3
orange scone, mini	1	160	29	2	1	4	2.5	15	150	1
pecan roll	1	730	87	5 ½	11	39	12.0	60	310	5
pumpkin muffin	1	580	89	6	7	22	4.0	30	470	2
shortbread cookie	1	350	36	2 ½	3	21	12.0	55	160	1
wild blueberry muffin	1	440	66	4 ½	6	17	3.0	60	330	2
wild blueberry scone	1	440	63	4	7	18	12.0	75	880	2
wild blueberry scone, mini	1	160	21	1 ½	2	6	4.0	25	290	1
Salads										
Asian sesame chicken	1	410	31	2	31	20	3.5	60	810	3
chopped chicken cobb	1	500	11	1	38	36	9.0	140	1130	3
Fuji apple chicken	1	520	36	2	32	31	7.0	80	830	5
Greek	1	380	14	1	8	34	8.0	20	1670	5
Sandwiches										
Asiago roast beef	1	760	64	4	49	27	14.0	100	1330	4
Bacon Turkey Bravo®	1	800	83	5 ½	52	29	10.0	85	2800	4
chicken Caesar	1	720	69	4 ½	43	32	10.0	130	1270	4
Italian combo	1	980	95	6	58	41	15.0	150	2620	5
Mediterranean veggie	1	600	98	6	22	13	3.5	10	1420	10
Napa almond chicken salad	1	690	90	6	29	26	4.5	60	1200	5
Sierra turkey	1	920	79	5	49	40	12.0	80	1900	4
smoked ham & Swiss	1	590	64	4	45	17	8.0	90	1870	5
smoked turkey	1	420	66	4 ½	33	3	0.5	30	1650	3
tuna salad	1	470	65	4	19	16	3.5	25	980	5
Soups										
broccoli cheddar	large	290	24	1	12	16	9.0	30	1540	7
cream of chicken & wild rice	large	310	60	4	10	17	8.0	60	1470	3
creamy tomato, w/ croutons	large	370	39	2 ½	4	23	12.0	15	740	5
French onion, w/ croutons	large	250	30	2	10	11	5.0	25	2380	3
low fat chicken noodle	large	140	23	1 ½	5	3	1.0	30	1450	0
low fat vegetable, w/ pesto	large	160	28	1 ½	5	4	0.0	0	1240	6
low fat vegetarian black bean	large	170	29	2	10	4	1.5	0	1590	5

FAST FOODS & RESTAURANT CHAINS
Pizza Hut®

ITEM	AMOUNT	CALORIES	CARBOHYDRATE (g)	CARBOHYDRATE CHOICES	PROTEIN (g)	FAT (g)	SATURATED FAT (g)	CHOLESTEROL (mg)	SODIUM (mg)	FIBER (g)
Pizza Hut®										
Breadstick, cheese, w/o dipping sauce	1	170	20	1	8	6	2.5	15	390	1
Buffalo wings, traditional										
hot	2	110	8	½	8	6	1.5	40	810	1
mild	2	110	8	½	8	6	1.5	40	830	1
Cheese pizza										
hand tossed	1 slice	220	26	2	10	8	4.0	25	550	1
pan	1 slice	240	27	2	11	10	4.5	25	530	1
Personal Pan®	1 pizza	590	69	4 ½	26	24	10.0	55	1290	3
Thin 'N Crispy®	1 slice	190	22	1 ½	9	8	4.0	25	550	1
Fit'n Delicious® pizza										
chicken, mushrooms & jalapeño	1 slice	170	22	1 ½	11	5	1.5	20	720	1
chicken, red onion & green pepper	1 slice	180	23	1 ½	11	5	1.5	20	510	1
diced red tomato, mushroom & jalapeño	1 slice	150	23	1 ½	6	4	1.5	10	610	2
green pepper, red onion & red tomato	1 slice	150	24	1 ½	6	4	1.5	10	400	2
ham, pineapple & diced red onions	1 slice	160	24	1 ½	7	5	1.5	15	550	1
Ham & pineapple pizza										
hand tossed	1 slice	200	27	2	9	6	3.0	20	550	1
pan	1 slice	230	28	2	10	9	3.5	20	520	1
Thin 'N Crispy®	1 slice	180	23	1 ½	8	6	3.0	20	540	1
Italian sausage & red onion										
hand tossed	1 slice	240	27	2	11	10	4.5	25	580	1
pan	1 slice	270	28	2	11	13	4.5	25	560	1
Thin 'N Crispy®	1 slice	220	23	1 ½	9	10	4.0	25	580	1
Meat Lover's® pizza										
hand tossed	1 slice	300	26	2	14	16	7.0	40	860	1
pan	1 slice	330	27	2	14	18	7.0	40	830	1
Personal Pan®	1 pizza	830	68	4 ½	36	46	17.0	100	2110	3
Thin 'N Crispy®	1 slice	280	22	1 ½	13	16	6.0	40	860	1
P'Zone®										
classic	½ order	470	61	4	20	16	7.0	40	1070	3
pepperoni	½ order	450	60	4	19	17	7.0	40	1120	2
Pepperoni pizza										
hand tossed	1 slice	230	25	1 ½	10	9	4.0	25	610	1
pan	1 slice	250	26	2	11	12	4.5	25	590	1
Personal Pan®	1 pizza	610	67	4 ½	26	26	10.0	55	1410	3
Thin 'N Crispy®	1 slice	200	21	1 ½	9	9	4.0	25	610	1
Stuffed pizza roller, w/o sauce	1	220	24	1 ½	9	10	4.5	25	580	1
Stuffed pizza roller dipping sauces										
marinara	3 oz.	60	12	1	2	0	0.0	0	440	2
ranch	1.5 oz.	220	2	0	0	23	3.5	10	420	0

FAST FOODS & RESTAURANT CHAINS
Pizza Hut®

ITEM	AMOUNT	CALORIES	CARBOHYDRATE (g)	CARBOHYDRATE CHOICES	PROTEIN (g)	FAT (g)	SATURATED FAT (g)	CHOLESTEROL (mg)	SODIUM (mg)	FIBER (g)
Supreme pizza										
hand tossed	1 slice	260	26	2	12	12	5.0	30	680	1
pan	1 slice	290	27	2	12	14	5.0	30	650	2
Thin 'N Crispy®	1 slice	240	23	1 ½	10	12	5.0	30	670	1
Tuscani pastas										
chicken Alfredo	½ pan	580	49	3	23	32	9.0	50	1250	4
meaty marinara	½ pan	450	44	3	20	20	8.0	70	1100	5
*Slice = 1/8 of 12-inch pie										

Starbuck's® Coffee Co.

ITEM	AMOUNT	CALORIES	CARBOHYDRATE (g)	CARBOHYDRATE CHOICES	PROTEIN (g)	FAT (g)	SATURATED FAT (g)	CHOLESTEROL (mg)	SODIUM (mg)	FIBER (g)
Bagels										
multigrain	1	160	31	2	6	2	0	0	110	2
plain	1	300	64	4	10	1	0	0	460	2
Bars										
blueberry oat	1	370	47	3	6	14	7.0	30	150	5
marshmallow dream	1	210	43	3	0	4	2.5	10	250	0
Brewed coffees, black										
coffee of the week	12 fl. oz.	5	0	0	0	0	0.0	0	10	0
decaf coffee of the week	12 fl. oz.	5	0	0	0	0	0.0	0	10	0
Caffé misto/café au lait										
w/ nonfat milk	12 fl. oz.	60	8	½	6	0	0.0	5	70	0
w/ whole milk	12 fl. oz.	100	7	½	5	5	3.0	15	65	0
Cakes										
banana nut loaf	1 piece	490	75	5	7	19	2.5	25	210	4
iced lemon pound	1 piece	490	68	4 ½	5	23	13.0	135	520	0
reduced-fat banana chocolate chip	1 piece	390	79	5	5	7	4.5	0	500	3
reduced-fat cinnamon swirl	1 piece	340	62	4	4	9	5.0	10	400	2
reduced-fat very berry	1 piece	350	59	4	7	10	4.0	60	490	4
Starbucks® classic coffee cake	1 piece	440	63	4	6	19	11.0	95	580	0
Classic favorite beverages										
apple juice	12 fl. oz.	190	48	3	0	0	0.0	0	20	0
apple juice, steamed	8 fl. oz.	110	43	3	0	0	0.0	0	15	0
hot chocolate, w/ whipped cream										
w/ nonfat milk	12 fl. oz.	250	39	2 ½	11	8	4.0	30	115	0
w/ soy milk	12 fl. oz.	280	42	2 ½	8	11	4.5	20	100	2
w/ whole milk	12 fl. oz.	320	38	2 ½	11	16	9.0	50	110	0
hot chocolate, w/o whipped cream										
w/ nonfat milk	12 fl. oz.	190	37	2 ½	11	2	0.0	0	110	0
w/ soy milk	12 fl. oz.	220	40	2 ½	8	5	1.0	0	95	2
w/ whole milk	12 fl. oz.	260	36	2 ½	10	10	5.0	25	105	0

FAST FOODS & RESTAURANT CHAINS
Starbucks® Coffee Co.

ITEM	AMOUNT	CALORIES	CARBOHYDRATE (g)	CARBOHYDRATE CHOICES	PROTEIN (g)	FAT (g)	SATURATED FAT (g)	CHOLESTEROL (mg)	SODIUM (mg)	FIBER (g)
milk										
nonfat	12 fl. oz.	140	20	1	14	0	0.0	10	170	0
soy	12 fl. oz.	190	25	1 ½	10	6	1.0	0	150	2
whole	12 fl. oz.	240	18	1	13	13	7.0	40	160	0
white hot chocolate, w/ whipped cream										
w/ nonfat milk	12 fl. oz.	330	49	3	12	10	7.0	30	200	0
w/ soy milk	12 fl. oz.	360	52	3 ½	9	14	8.0	25	190	0
w/ whole milk	12 fl. oz.	400	47	3	12	19	12.0	50	200	0
white hot chocolate, w/o whipped cream										
w/ nonfat milk	12 fl. oz.	270	47	3	12	5	3.5	0	200	0
w/ soy milk	12 fl. oz.	300	50	3	9	8	3.5	0	180	0
w/ whole milk	12 fl. oz.	340	46	3	12	13	8.0	30	190	0
Cookies										
chocolate chunk	1	380	51	3 ½	4	17	10.0	65	230	2
outrageous oatmeal	1	370	56	4	5	14	8.0	65	170	3
treat-sized peanut butter	1	160	20	1	3	8	3.0	20	100	2
treat-sized double chocolate	1	130	16	1	2	8	4.5	25	35	0
Croissants										
butter	1	310	32	2	5	18	11.0	45	290	0
chocolate	1	300	34	2	5	17	10.0	30	220	2
Espresso, hot										
caffè Americano	12 fl. oz.	10	2	0	0	0	0.0	0	5	0
caffè latte										
w/ nonfat milk	12 fl. oz.	100	15	1	10	0	0.0	0	120	0
w/ soy milk	12 fl. oz.	130	18	1	7	4	0.5	0	100	0
w/ whole milk	12 fl. oz.	180	14	1	10	9	5.0	30	115	0
caffè mocha, w/ whipped cream										
w/ nonfat milk	12 fl. oz.	230	34	2	11	8	4.0	25	110	0
w/ soy milk	12 fl. oz.	260	36	2 ½	8	11	4.5	20	95	2
w/ whole milk	12 fl. oz.	290	33	2	10	15	9.0	45	105	0
caffè mocha, w/o whipped cream										
w/ nonfat milk	12 fl. oz.	170	32	2	10	2	0.0	0	100	0
w/ soy milk	12 fl. oz.	190	34	2	8	5	0.5	0	90	2
w/ whole milk	12 fl. oz.	230	31	2	10	9	4.5	25	100	0
cappuccino										
w/ nonfat milk	12 fl. oz.	60	9	½	6	0	0.0	0	70	0
w/ soy milk	12 fl. oz.	80	11	1	4	3	0.0	0	60	0
w/ whole milk	12 fl. oz.	110	9	½	6	6	3.0	15	70	0
caramel macchiato										
w/ nonfat milk	12 fl. oz.	140	25	1 ½	8	1	0.5	0	105	0
w/ soy milk	12 fl. oz.	170	28	2	6	4	1.0	0	90	0
w/ whole milk	12 fl. oz.	200	24	1 ½	8	8	4.5	25	100	0

Starbucks® Coffee Co.

ITEM	AMOUNT	CALORIES	CARBOHYDRATE (g)	CARBOHYDRATE CHOICES	PROTEIN (g)	FAT (g)	SATURATED FAT (g)	CHOLESTEROL (mg)	SODIUM (mg)	FIBER (g)
Espresso, iced										
iced caffè Americano	12 fl. oz.	10	2	0	0	0	0.0	0	5	0
iced caffè latte										
w/ nonfat milk	12 fl. oz.	70	10	½	6	0	0.0	0	80	0
w/ soy milk	12 fl. oz.	90	13	1	5	3	0.0	0	70	0
w/ whole milk	12 fl. oz.	110	9	½	6	6	3.5	20	75	0
iced caffè mocha, w/ whipped cream										
w/ nonfat milk	12 fl. oz.	210	29	2	7	10	5.0	30	70	0
w/ soy milk	12 fl. oz.	230	31	2	6	12	6.0	30	65	2
w/ whole milk	12 fl. oz.	250	28	2	7	14	8.0	45	70	0
iced caffè mocha, w/o whipped cream										
w/ nonfat milk	12 fl. oz.	130	27	2	7	2	0.0	0	65	0
w/ soy milk	12 fl. oz.	150	28	2	5	4	0.5	0	55	2
w/ whole milk	12 fl. oz.	170	26	2	7	6	3.0	15	60	0
iced caramel macchiato										
w/ nonfat milk	12 fl. oz.	140	25	1 ½	7	1	1.0	0	100	0
w/ soy milk	12 fl. oz.	170	28	2	5	4	1.0	0	90	0
w/ whole milk	12 fl. oz.	190	24	1 ½	7	7	4.5	35	95	0
Frappucino® blended beverages										
caramel, w/ whipped cream										
w/ nonfat milk	12 fl. oz.	270	45	3	3	9	5.0	35	170	0
w/ whole milk	12 fl. oz.	290	45	3	3	11	7.0	40	160	0
caramel, w/o whipped cream										
w/ nonfat milk	12 fl. oz.	170	40	2 ½	3	0	0.0	0	150	0
w/ whole milk	12 fl. oz.	190	40	2 ½	3	3	1.5	10	150	0
coconut crème, w/ whipped cream										
w/ nonfat milk	12 fl. oz.	230	34	2	4	9	6.0	30	170	0
w/ whole milk	12 fl. oz.	260	34	2	4	12	7.0	40	170	0
coconut crème, w/o whipped cream										
w/ nonfat milk	12 fl. oz.	140	31	2	4	0	0.0	0	160	0
w/ whole milk	12 fl. oz.	170	31	2	3	4	2.0	10	160	0
coffee, light blended	12 fl. oz.	110	27	2	3	0	0.0	0	200	0
coffee, regular blend, w/o whipped cream										
w/ nonfat milk	12 fl. oz.	160	36	2 ½	3	0	0.0	0	160	0
w/ soy milk	12 fl. oz.	170	37	2 ½	2	2	0.0	0	150	0
w/ whole milk	12 fl. oz.	180	36	2 ½	3	3	1.5	10	150	0
vanilla bean, w/ whipped cream										
w/ nonfat milk	12 fl. oz.	250	42	3	4	8	5.0	30	170	0
w/ soy milk	12 fl. oz.	270	43	3	3	10	5.0	30	170	0
w/ whole milk	12 fl. oz.	280	41	3	4	12	7.0	40	170	0
vanilla bean, w/o whipped cream										
w/ nonfat milk	12 fl. oz.	170	40	2 ½	4	0	0.0	0	160	0

FAST FOODS & RESTAURANT CHAINS

Starbucks® Coffee Co.

ITEM	AMOUNT	CALORIES	CARBOHYDRATE (g)	CARBOHYDRATE CHOICES	PROTEIN (g)	FAT (g)	SATURATED FAT (g)	CHOLESTEROL (mg)	SODIUM (mg)	FIBER (g)
Frappucino® blended beverages, vanilla bean w/o whipped cream *(continued)*										
w/ soy milk	12 fl. oz.	190	41	3	3	2	0.0	0	160	0
w/ whole milk	12 fl. oz.	200	39	2 ½	3	4	2.0	10	160	0
Iced shaken refreshments										
iced shaken coffee	12 fl. oz.	60	15	1	0	0	0.0	0	0	0
Tazo® green iced tea	12 fl. oz.	60	16	1	0	0	0.0	0	10	0
Muffins										
apple bran	1	350	64	4	6	9	2.5	65	520	7
blueberry streusel	1	360	59	4	7	11	6.0	80	390	2
lowfat red raspberry	1	340	65	1 ½	7	6	1.5	50	500	2
Petite bakery items										
birthday mini doughnut	1	130	17	1	0	6	2.5	10	140	0
carrot cake mini cupcake	1	190	21	1 ½	0	11	5.0	25	140	0
double fudge mini doughnut	1	130	16	1	0	7	3.0	0	170	0
red velvet whoopie pie	1	190	21	1 ½	0	11	5.0	20	180	0
rocky road cake pop	1	180	23	1 ½	3	9	5.0	10	80	0
tiramisu cake pop	1	170	22	1 ½	0	9	5.0	10	90	0
vanilla scone	1	140	21	1 ½	0	5	2.5	15	90	0
Scones										
blueberry	1	460	61	4	7	22	12.0	75	420	2
cranberry orange	1	490	73	5	8	18	9.0	55	460	2
maple oat pecan	1	440	59	4	8	18	11.0	75	490	3
Sweet rolls, Danishes & bars										
apple fritter	1	420	59	4	5	20	9.0	0	360	0
blueberry oat bar	1	370	47	2 ½	6	14	7.0	30	150	5
cheese Danish	1	420	39	2 ½	7	25	16.0	115	370	0
Mallorca sweet bread	1	420	42	3	7	25	12.0	200	600	0
Tazo® teas										
chai latte, hot										
w/ nonfat milk	12 fl. oz.	150	33	2	6	0	0.0	0	75	0
w/ soy milk	12 fl. oz.	170	35	2	4	2	0.0	0	65	0
w/ whole milk	12 fl. oz.	200	33	2	6	5	3.0	15	70	0
iced green tea latte										
w/ nonfat milk	12 fl. oz.	160	32	2	7	0	0.0	0	85	0
w/ soy milk	12 fl. oz.	190	35	2	5	3	0.0	0	80	2
w/ whole milk	12 fl. oz.	210	31	2	7	7	3.5	20	85	0
Vivanno™ smoothie, chocolate										
w/ 2% milk	16 fl. oz.	250	48	3	18	5	2.5	15	140	6
w/ nonfat milk	16 fl. oz.	250	48	3	18	2	0.5	0	140	6
w/ soy milk	16 fl. oz.	270	50	3	17	4	0.5	0	135	7
Warm breakfast items										
bacon, gouda & egg frittata on artisan bread	1	350	30	2	17	18	7.0	170	840	0

FAST FOODS & RESTAURANT CHAINS

Starbucks® Coffee Co.

ITEM	AMOUNT	CALORIES	CARBOHYDRATE (g)	CARBOHYDRATE CHOICES	PROTEIN (g)	FAT (g)	SATURATED FAT (g)	CHOLESTEROL (mg)	SODIUM (mg)	FIBER (g)
Warm breakfast items *(continued)*										
egg white, spinach & feta wrap	1	280	33	2	18	10	3.5	20	900	6
perfect oatmeal toppings										
brown sugar	1 side	50	13	1	0	0	0.0	0	0	0
dried fruit	1 side	100	24	1 ½	0	0	0.0	0	10	2
nut medley	1 side	100	2	0	2	9	1.0	0	0	0
perfect oatmeal, w/o toppings	1 serving	140	25	1 ½	5	3	0.5	0	105	4
reduced-fat turkey bacon,										
egg white & cheese on English muffin	1	320	43	3	18	7	2.0	20	700	3
sausage, egg & cheddar on English muffin	1	500	41	3	19	28	9.0	185	1000	0

Subway®

ITEM	AMOUNT	CALORIES	CARBOHYDRATE (g)	CARBOHYDRATE CHOICES	PROTEIN (g)	FAT (g)	SATURATED FAT (g)	CHOLESTEROL (mg)	SODIUM (mg)	FIBER (g)
Breads										
9-grain wheat	1 (6 inch)	210	40	2 ½	8	2	0.5	0	310	4
flatbread	1 (3 oz.)	220	38	2 ½	7	5	1.0	0	450	2
honey oat	1 (6 inch)	260	48	3	9	3	0.5	0	330	5
Italian herbs & cheese	1 (6 inch)	250	40	2 ½	9	5	2.5	10	490	2
Italian white bread	1 (6 inch)	200	38	2 ½	7	2	0.5	0	290	1
mini Italian, white	1 (1.7 oz.)	130	25	1 ½	5	2	0.0	0	190	1
mini wheat	1 (1.8 oz.)	140	27	2	5	2	0.0	0	200	3
Monterey cheddar	1 (6 inch)	240	38	2 ½	10	6	2.5	10	360	2
parmesan oregano	1 (6 inch)	220	40	2 ½	8	3	1.0	0	440	2
roasted garlic	1 (6 inch)	230	45	3	8	3	0.5	0	1260	2
sourdough	1 (6 inch)	210	41	3	8	3	1.0	0	210	3
Condiments & extras										
American cheese	2 triangles	40	1	0	2	4	2.0	10	200	0
bacon	2 strips	45	0	0	3	4	1.5	10	190	0
mayonnaise, light	1 T.	50	0	0	0	5	1.0	5	100	0
mayonnaise, regular	1 T.	110	0	0	0	12	2.0	10	80	0
Desserts & cookies										
chocolate chip	1 order	210	30	2	2	10	6.0	15	150	1
chocolate chunk	1 order	200	30	2	2	10	5.0	10	100	1
double chocolate	1 order	210	30	2	2	10	5.0	15	170	1
M & M	1 order	210	32	2	2	10	5.0	10	100	1
oatmeal raisin	1 order	200	30	2	3	8	4.0	15	170	1
peanut butter	1 order	220	26	2	4	12	5.0	15	200	1
raspberry cheesecake	1 order	210	29	2	2	9	4.5	15	160	0
sugar	1 order	220	28	2	2	12	6.0	15	140	0
white macadamia nut	1 order	220	29	2	2	11	5.0	15	160	1
Egg muffin melts										
bacon, egg & cheese	1	200	24	1 ½	13	7	3.0	120	550	6
egg & cheese	1	170	24	1 ½	12	6	2.0	115	460	6

FAST FOODS & RESTAURANT CHAINS

Subway®

ITEM	AMOUNT	CALORIES	CARBOHYDRATE (g)	CARBOHYDRATE CHOICES	PROTEIN (g)	FAT (g)	SATURATED FAT (g)	CHOLESTEROL (mg)	SODIUM (mg)	FIBER (g)
Egg muffin melts *(continued)*										
Sunrise Subway®	1	230	26	1 ½	18	8	3.0	130	810	6
Egg white muffin melts										
Breakfast BMT® melt, w/ egg white	1	220	25	1 ½	16	8	3.0	20	860	5
egg white & cheese, w/ ham	1	170	24	1 ½	14	4	1.5	10	610	5
Sunrise Subway®	1	210	26	1 ½	18	6	2.5	20	830	5
Fruizle Express										
berry lishus	small	110	28	2	1	0	0.0	0	30	1
peach pizazz	small	100	26	2	0	0	0.0	0	25	0
sunrise refresher	small	120	29	2	1	0	0.0	0	20	1
Omelet sandwiches										
bacon, egg & cheese	1 (6 inch)	410	45	3	23	16	6.0	235	1080	5
Breakfast BMT®	1 (6 inch)	500	47	3	29	22	8.0	265	1640	5
Sunrise Subway®	1 (6 inch)	470	48	3	32	17	7.0	260	1600	5
Salad dressings										
fat free Italian	2 oz.	35	7	½	1	0	0.0	0	720	0
ranch	2 oz.	320	3	0	0	35	6.0	30	560	0
Salads, w/ 6 grams of fat or less										
ham	1	110	11	1	12	3	1.0	20	590	4
oven roasted chicken	1	130	9	½	19	3	0.5	50	270	4
roast beef	1	140	10	½	18	4	1.0	40	450	4
Subway Club®	1	140	11	1	17	4	1.0	40	640	4
turkey breast	1	110	11	1	12	2	0.5	20	570	4
turkey breast & ham	1	110	11	1	12	3	0.5	25	580	4
Veggie Delite®	1	50	9	½	3	1	0.0	0	65	4
Sandwiches, cold										
orchard chicken salad	1 (6 inch)	370	54	3 ½	20	8	1.5	40	560	6
tuna	1 (6 inch)	530	44	3	21	30	6.0	45	830	5
Sandwiches, flatbread										
black forest ham	1	300	44	3	17	7	1.5	25	980	3
roast beef	1	330	43	3	23	7	2.0	40	840	3
roasted chicken breast	1	330	45	3	22	7	1.5	25	790	3
Subway Club®	1	320	44	3	23	7	2.0	40	1030	3
sweet onion chicken teriyaki	1	390	57	4	25	7	1.5	50	1050	3
turkey breast	1	290	44	3	17	6	1.5	20	950	3
turkey breast & ham	1	290	44	3	17	6	1.5	25	960	3
Veggie Delite®	1	240	42	3	8	5	1.0	0	450	3
Sandwiches, lowfat footlong										
ham	1 (12 inch)	570	92	6	35	9	2.5	50	1670	10
oven roasted chicken	1 (12 inch)	640	95	6	46	10	2.5	45	1290	11
roast beef	1 (12 inch)	630	90	5 ½	48	10	3.5	90	1390	11
Subway Club®	1 (12 inch)	630	92	6	46	9	3.0	80	1770	10

ITEM	AMOUNT	CALORIES	CARBOHYDRATE (g)	CARBOHYDRATE CHOICES	PROTEIN (g)	FAT (g)	SATURATED FAT (g)	CHOLESTEROL (mg)	SODIUM (mg)	FIBER (g)
Sandwiches, lowfat footlong *(continued)*										
sweet onion chicken teriyaki	1 (12 inch)	750	117	7 ½	51	9	2.5	100	1810	10
turkey breast	1 (12 inch)	560	92	6	35	7	2.0	40	1620	10
turkey breast & ham	1 (12 inch)	570	92	6	35	8	2.0	45	1650	10
Veggie Delite®	1 (12 inch)	460	87	5 ½	17	5	1.0	0	620	10
Sandwiches, mini subs										
ham	1	180	30	2	10	3	0.5	10	470	3
roast beef	1	200	30	2	14	3	1.0	25	410	4
turkey breast	1	180	30	2	10	2	0.5	10	460	3
Veggie Delite®	1	150	29	2	6	2	0.0	0	210	3
Sandwiches, toasted										
cheesesteak	1 (6 inch)	520	52	3	39	18	9.0	90	1370	6
BLT	1 (6 inch)	360	44	3	17	13	6.0	30	890	5
Buffalo chicken	1 (6 inch)	420	46	3	25	15	3.0	55	1190	5
chicken & bacon ranch	1 (6 inch)	570	47	3	35	28	10.0	95	1080	5
feast	1 (6 inch)	550	51	3	39	23	9.0	85	2610	6
Italian B.M.T.®	1 (6 inch)	450	47	3	22	20	8.0	55	1500	5
meatball marinara	1 (6 inch)	580	69	4	24	23	9.0	45	1420	9
spicy Italian	1 (6 inch)	520	46	3	22	28	11.0	65	1720	5
steak and cheese	1 (6 inch)	380	48	3	26	10	4.5	50	1060	5
Subway Melt®	1 (6 inch)	370	47	3	23	11	5.0	45	1210	5
Sandwiches, w/ 6 grams of fat or less										
black forest ham, w/o cheese	1 (6 inch)	290	46	3	18	5	1.0	20	830	5
oven roasted chicken	1 (6 inch)	320	47	3	23	5	1.5	25	640	5
roast beef	1 (6 inch)	320	45	3	24	5	1.5	40	700	5
Subway Club®	1 (6 inch)	310	46	3	23	5	1.5	40	880	5
sweet onion chicken teriyaki	1 (6 inch)	380	59	4	26	5	1.0	50	900	5
turkey breast	1 (6 inch)	280	46	3	18	4	1.0	20	810	5
turkey breast & ham	1 (6 inch)	300	46	3	19	4	1.0	25	910	5
Veggie Delite®	1 (6 inch)	230	44	3	8	3	0.5	0	310	5
Soups										
chicken & dumpling	1 bowl	170	23	1 ½	8	5	2.0	35	810	2
chicken tortilla	1 bowl	110	11	1	6	2	0.5	10	440	3
chili con carne	1 bowl	340	35	2	20	11	5.0	60	950	10
chipotle chicken corn chowder	1 bowl	140	22	1 ½	6	3	1.5	15	900	2
cream of potato, w/ bacon	1 bowl	240	26	2	5	13	5.0	15	870	3
fire-roasted tomato orzo	1 bowl	130	24	1 ½	6	1	0.5	5	410	2
golden broccoli & cheese	1 bowl	180	16	1	5	11	5.0	25	990	4
minestrone	1 bowl	90	17	1	4	1	0.0	0	910	3
New England clam chowder	1 bowl	150	20	1	6	5	1.0	10	990	2
roasted chicken noodle	1 bowl	80	12	1	6	2	0.5	15	950	1
Rosemary chicken & dumpling	1 bowl	90	14	1	6	2	0.5	25	810	1

ITEM	AMOUNT	CALORIES	CARBOHYDRATE (g)	CARBOHYDRATE CHOICES	PROTEIN (g)	FAT (g)	SATURATED FAT (g)	CHOLESTEROL (mg)	SODIUM (mg)	FIBER (g)
Soups *(continued)*										
Spanish style chicken & rice	1 bowl	110	16	1	6	3	1.0	5	980	1
tomato garden vegetable, w/ rotini	1 bowl	90	20	1	3	1	0.0	0	820	3
vegetable beef	1 bowl	100	17	1	5	2	0.5	10	960	3
wild rice, w/ chicken	1 bowl	230	26	2	6	11	3.5	50	900	1
(Subs, salads & sandwiches do not include cheese, mayonnaise, oil or sauce unless specified).										
Taco Bell®										
Drinks										
cherry limeade sparkler	16 oz.	180	43	3	0	0	0.0	0	105	0
cherry limeade sparkler	20 oz.	270	66	4 ½	0	0	0.0	0	160	0
classic limeade sparkler	16 oz.	150	39	2 ½	0	0	0.0	0	80	0
classic limeade sparkler	20 oz.	230	60	4	0	0	0.0	0	125	0
Mango Strawberry Frutista Freeze®	16 oz.	250	62	4	0	0	0.0	0	10	0
Strawberry Frutista Freeze®	16 oz.	230	57	4	0	0	0.0	0	55	0
Burritos										
½ lb. cheesy potato	1	540	59	3 ½	19	26	8.0	50	1430	7
½ lb. combo	1	460	53	3	21	18	7.0	50	1400	10
7-layer	1	500	69	4	17	18	6.0	20	1090	12
bean	1	370	56	3 ½	13	10	3.5	5	980	10
beefy 5-layer	1	540	68	4	19	21	8.0	35	1320	9
beefy crunch	1	500	61	4	15	22	6.0	30	1090	5
Burrito Supreme®, beef	1	420	53	3	17	15	7.0	35	1140	9
Burrito Supreme®, chicken	1	400	51	3	21	12	5.0	40	1060	7
Burrito Supreme®, steak	1	390	51	3	17	13	5.0	30	1100	7
cheesy bean & rice	1	480	60	4	12	21	5.0	10	1030	7
cheesy double beef	1	470	54	3 ½	18	20	6.0	45	1270	6
chili cheese	1	380	41	2 ½	16	17	8.0	35	930	5
fresco bean	1	350	57	3 ½	12	8	2.5	0	990	11
grilled chicken	1	430	48	3	18	18	5.0	35	870	3
grilled stuft, beef	1	700	79	5	27	30	10.0	60	1740	12
grilled stuft, chicken	1	650	76	5	34	24	7.0	65	1580	9
grilled stuft, steak	1	640	76	5	28	25	8.0	50	1670	9
Chalupas										
Baja, beef	1	410	30	2	13	26	5.0	35	690	5
Baja, chicken	1	390	28	2	16	23	4.0	35	610	3
Baja, steak	1	380	28	2	13	23	4.0	30	650	3
nacho cheese, beef	1	360	31	2	11	21	3.5	20	660	4
nacho cheese, chicken	1	340	30	2	15	18	2.0	25	580	3
nacho cheese, steak	1	330	30	2	12	19	2.5	20	620	3
supreme, beef	1	370	31	2	13	21	5.0	35	600	4
supreme, chicken	1	350	29	2	17	18	4.0	35	520	3

ITEM	AMOUNT	CALORIES	CARBOHYDRATE (g)	CARBOHYDRATE CHOICES	PROTEIN (g)	FAT (g)	SATURATED FAT (g)	CHOLESTEROL (mg)	SODIUM (mg)	FIBER (g)
Chalupas *(continued)*										
supreme, steak	1	340	29	2	14	18	4.0	30	570	3
Condiments & sauces										
avocado ranch dressing	1 serving	80	1	0	0	8	1.5	5	50	0
border sauce, fire	1 serving	0	0	0	0	0	0.0	0	60	0
border sauce, hot	1 serving	0	0	0	0	0	0.0	0	45	0
border sauce, mild	1 serving	0	0	0	0	0	0.0	0	35	0
creamy jalapeño sauce	1 serving	70	1	0	0	7	1.0	5	50	0
fiesta salsa	1 serving	5	1	0	0	0	0.0	0	60	1
fire roasted salsa	1 serving	0	1	0	0	0	0.0	0	45	0
green tomatillo sauce	1 serving	10	2	0	0	0	0.0	0	170	0
guacamole	1 serving	35	2	0	0	3	0.0	0	85	1
pepper jack sauce	1 serving	70	1	0	0	7	1.0	5	50	0
pizza sauce	1 serving	10	2	0	0	0	0.0	0	90	0
red sauce	1 serving	10	2	0	0	0	0.0	0	170	0
reduced fat sour cream	1 serving	30	2	0	1	2	1.0	5	20	0
salsa	1 serving	5	1	0	0	0	0.0	0	80	0
salsa verde	1 serving	0	1	0	0	0	0.0	0	55	0
zesty dressing	1 serving	200	3	0	1	20	3.5	0	250	0
Fresco menu										
bean burrito	1	350	57	3 ½	12	8	2.5	0	990	11
Burrito Supreme®, chicken	1	350	50	3	18	8	2.5	25	1060	7
Burrito Supreme®, steak	1	340	50	3	15	8	2.5	15	1100	7
chicken soft taco	1	150	18	1	12	4	1.0	25	480	2
crunchy taco	1	150	13	1	7	7	2.5	20	350	3
grilled steak soft taco	1	150	19	1	9	4	1.5	15	520	2
soft taco	1	180	20	1	8	7	2.5	20	560	3
Gorditas										
Gordita Baja®, beef	1	340	30	2	13	18	5.0	35	680	4
Gordita Baja®, chicken	1	310	28	2	17	15	3.5	35	600	3
Gordita Baja®, steak	1	310	28	2	14	15	3.5	30	640	3
Gordita Supreme®, beef	1	300	31	2	13	13	5.0	35	590	4
Gordita Supreme®, chicken	1	270	29	2	17	10	3.5	35	510	2
Gordita Supreme®, steak	1	270	29	2	14	11	4.0	30	550	2
nacho cheese, beef	1	290	31	2	12	14	3.0	20	650	4
nacho cheese, chicken	1	270	29	2	15	10	1.5	25	570	2
nacho cheese, steak	1	260	29	2	12	11	2.0	20	610	2
Nachos										
cheesy	1 order	280	28	2	3	17	1.5	0	230	2
Nachos BellGrande®	1 order	770	79	5	19	42	7.0	30	1050	14
plain	1 order	330	31	2	4	20	2.0	5	370	2
supreme	1 order	440	42	2 ½	12	24	5.0	30	680	8

FAST FOODS & RESTAURANT CHAINS
Taco Bell®

ITEM	AMOUNT	CALORIES	CARBOHYDRATE (g)	CARBOHYDRATE CHOICES	PROTEIN (g)	FAT (g)	SATURATED FAT (g)	CHOLESTEROL (mg)	SODIUM (mg)	FIBER (g)
Nachos *(continued)*										
volcano	1 order	980	89	5 ½	21	60	9.0	45	1620	15
Sides										
caramel apple empanada	1 side	310	39	2 ½	3	15	2.5	0	310	2
cheesy fiesta potatoes	1 side	270	28	2	4	16	2.5	10	770	3
cinnamon twists	1 side	170	26	2	1	7	0.0	0	200	1
Mexican rice	1 side	120	20	1	2	4	0.0	0	200	1
pintos 'n cheese	1 side	170	20	1	9	6	3.0	10	580	8
Specialties										
cheese quesadilla	1	480	40	2 ½	19	27	11.0	50	1000	4
cheese roll-up	1	190	18	1	9	9	5.0	20	450	2
chicken quesadilla	1	530	41	3	28	28	12.0	75	1210	4
chili cheese burrito	1	380	41	2 ½	16	17	8.0	35	930	5
Crunchwrap Supreme®	1	540	71	4 ½	17	21	7.0	30	1150	7
Enchirito®, beef	1	360	34	2	18	17	8.0	45	1160	8
Enchirito®, chicken	1	340	32	2	22	14	7.0	50	1080	6
Enchirito®, steak	1	330	32	2	19	14	7.0	45	1120	6
express taco salad, w/ chips	1	580	59	3 ½	23	28	10.0	60	1350	9
grilled chicken taquitos	1	320	37	2 ½	18	11	4.5	40	770	3
grilled steak taquitos	1	310	37	2 ½	15	11	5.0	30	810	3
Mexican pizza	1	540	47	3	20	30	8.0	45	980	8
MexiMelt®	1	270	21	1 ½	15	14	7.0	45	800	4
steak quesadilla	1	520	41	3	25	28	12.0	65	1250	4
tostada	1	250	30	1 ½	10	10	3.5	15	550	9
Taco salads										
chicken ranch	1	910	69	4	34	55	10.0	70	1200	8
chipotle steak	1	900	69	4	27	57	11.0	65	1480	8
express, w/ chips	1	580	59	3 ½	23	28	10.0	60	1350	9
fiesta	1	770	74	4 ½	26	42	10.0	60	1420	12
Tacos										
Cheesy Double Decker®	1	350	39	2	14	15	5.0	30	760	8
chicken, soft	1	180	18	1	14	6	2.5	30	460	1
crispy potato, soft	1	270	31	2	6	13	3.0	10	520	3
crunchy	1	170	12	1	8	10	3.5	30	330	3
Double Decker®	1	320	37	2	13	13	4.5	30	690	8
Double Decker® Taco Supreme®	1	350	40	2 ½	14	15	6.0	35	710	8
fresco, crunchy	1	150	13	1	7	7	2.5	20	350	3
fresco chicken, soft	1	150	18	1	12	4	1.0	25	480	2
grilled steak, soft	1	250	19	1	11	14	4.0	30	550	2
soft, beef	1	210	21	1 ½	10	9	4.0	30	560	3
Soft Taco Supreme®, beef	1	230	22	1 ½	11	11	5.0	35	560	3
Taco Supreme®	1	200	15	1	9	12	5.0	35	350	3

Uno® Chicago Grill

ITEM	AMOUNT	CALORIES	CARBOHYDRATE (g)	CARBOHYDRATE CHOICES	PROTEIN (g)	FAT (g)	SATURATED FAT (g)	CHOLESTEROL (mg)	SODIUM (mg)	FIBER (g)
Appetizers										
Buffalo wings	⅓ order	450	4	0	22	36	8.0	145	1180	0
calamari	⅓ order	350	28	2	13	31	3.5	130	690	1
crispy cheese dippers	⅓ order	280	27	2	12	16	6.0	35	830	1
shrimp & crab fondue	⅓ order	220	13	1	8	16	4.5	55	500	0
Chicken dishes, w/o breadsticks or sides										
baked stuffed	½ order	180	3	0	27	9	3.0	60	610	1
Chicken Thumb Platter®	½ order	240	17	1	27	9	1.5	60	790	1
herb rubbed breast	½ order	260	1	0	20	21	2.5	50	630	0
Milanese	½ order	430	21	1 ½	28	29	5.0	60	1120	3
Romano crusted parmesan	½ order	560	69	4 ½	37	19	4.5	65	1270	5
Deep dish pizza										
cheese & tomato, individual	⅓ pizza	580	39	2 ½	21	40	12.0	35	830	2
cheese & tomato, regular	1/6 pizza	580	39	2 ½	21	40	12.0	35	830	2
classic Chicago, individual	⅓ pizza	770	40	2 ½	33	55	18.0	75	1550	2
classic Chicago, regular	1/6 pizza	770	40	2 ½	33	55	18.0	75	1550	2
farmer's market vegetable, individual	⅓ pizza	540	42	3	15	35	9.0	20	750	3
farmer's market vegetable, regular	1/6 pizza	540	42	3	15	35	9.0	20	750	3
Numero Uno®, individual	⅓ pizza	640	41	3	21	44	12.0	45	1170	2
Numero Uno®, regular	1/6 pizza	640	41	3	21	44	12.0	45	1170	2
prima pepperoni, individual	⅓ pizza	610	39	2 ½	20	42	12.0	40	970	2
prima pepperoni, regular	1/6 pizza	610	39	2 ½	20	42	12.0	40	970	2
Spinoccolli®, individual	⅓ pizza	620	40	2 ½	16	45	11.0	20	780	3
Spinoccolli®, regular	1/6 pizza	620	40	2 ½	16	45	11.0	20	780	3
Desserts										
all American	½ order	330	45	3	3	15	8.0	50	260	3
bananas foster	½ order	640	82	5 ½	8	32	18.0	90	260	2
brownie bowl	½ order	430	57	4	4	20	12.0	60	220	2
mini chocolate peanut butter cup	1 order	360	35	2	5	22	11.0	35	150	2
mini hot chocolate brownie sundae	1 order	370	54	3 ½	4	16	8.0	60	190	2
Fish dishes										
baked haddock	½ order	290	6	½	27	17	3.0	70	270	0
Cajun blackened salmon	½ order	310	5	0	22	22	5.0	75	500	1
fish & chips	½ order	460	36	2	21	35	4.5	60	860	5
lemon basil salmon	½ order	240	0	0	21	17	2.5	60	370	0
Pasta dishes, w/o breadsticks										
chicken broccoli, w/ lemon pesto	½ order	650	48	3	26	49	7.0	45	740	4
Chicken Spinoccoli®	½ order	650	57	4	41	31	13.0	115	1330	4
chicken & broccoli Alfredo	½ order	620	53	3 ½	28	35	11.0	85	820	3

FAST FOODS & RESTAURANT CHAINS

Uno® Chicago Grill

ITEM	AMOUNT	CALORIES	CARBOHYDRATE (g)	CARBOHYDRATE CHOICES	PROTEIN (g)	FAT (g)	SATURATED FAT (g)	CHOLESTEROL (mg)	SODIUM (mg)	FIBER (g)
Pasta dishes, w/o breadsticks *(continued)*										
rattlesnake pasta	½ order	640	52	3 ½	29	37	12.0	95	910	3
shrimp scampi	½ order	580	53	3 ½	22	32	12.0	125	970	3
Salad dressings										
avocado ranch	1 serving	200	6	½	1	20	3.0	20	350	1
Caesar	1 serving	290	2	0	4	29	6.0	35	440	0
classic vinaigrete	1 serving	170	5	0	0	16	2.5	0	190	0
fat free vinaigrete	1 serving	30	5	0	0	0	0.0	0	200	0
Salads, large										
chopped honey crisp chicken	½ order	480	30	2	26	31	8.0	75	930	3
chopped power	½ order	270	32	2	23	7	1.5	45	610	5
classic cobb	½ order	440	11	½	26	34	10.0	210	1080	5
walnut crusted goat cheese	½ order	250	17	1	2	17	6.0	30	210	2
Sandwiches, w/o sides										
grilled chicken	1	300	23	1 ½	31	11	1.0	100	870	2
roasted vegetable & goat cheese wrap	1	210	23	1	11	10	3.0	10	460	6
Uno Burger®	1	390	14	1	22	27	10.0	105	690	1
veggie burger	1	200	22	1 ½	13	8	1.0	20	1130	4
Sides										
Farro salad	1	90	8	½	1	6	1.0	0	310	1
French fries	1 order	450	36	2	5	33	4.5	0	1290	7
red bliss mashed potatoes	1 order	270	34	2	4	14	3.5	5	650	3
rice pilaf	1 order	220	38	2 ½	5	6	1.5	0	340	1
roasted seasonal vegetables	1 order	100	13	1	2	5	0.0	0	115	3
smashed cauliflower	1 order	130	9	½	9	23	6.0	15	630	4
steamed seasonal vegetables	1 order	80	10	½	2	5	0.0	0	160	3
whole grain brown rice	1 order	180	32	2	3	6	0.5	0	100	1
Soups, w/o crackers										
chili	1 cup	270	36	2	14	8	3.5	30	830	7
Italian wedding	1 cup	120	16	1	6	4	1.0	15	730	2
New England clam chowder	1 cup	280	21	1 ½	9	18	10.0	70	780	1
Tuscan pesto minestrone	1 cup	100	16	1	4	2	0.0	0	930	3
veggie	1 cup	90	18	1	4	1	0.0	0	620	3
Steak dishes, w/o breadsticks or sides										
brewmasters grill NY sirloin	½ order	260	12	1	43	7	2.5	90	790	0
sirloin tips	½ order	290	4	0	31	14	4.0	85	1030	1
top sirloin	½ order	200	0	0	33	7	2.5	50	660	0
Traditional thin crust										
BBQ chicken	⅓ pizza	340	39	2 ½	18	12	5.0	40	660	1
cheese & tomato	⅓ pizza	280	33	2	11	11	5.0	20	590	1
four cheese	⅓ pizza	360	34	2	14	18	8.0	35	710	2
harvest vegetable	⅓ pizza	290	38	2 ½	9	11	3.5	15	560	4

FAST FOODS & RESTAURANT CHAINS

Uno® Chicago Grill

ITEM	AMOUNT	CALORIES	CARBOHYDRATE (g)	CARBOHYDRATE CHOICES	PROTEIN (g)	FAT (g)	SATURATED FAT (g)	CHOLESTEROL (mg)	SODIUM (mg)	FIBER (g)
Traditional thin crust *(continued)*										
Mediterranean	⅓ pizza	310	32	2	9	16	5.0	15	800	2
pepperoni	⅓ pizza	330	33	2	13	16	7.0	30	780	1
roasted eggplant, spinach & mushroom	⅓ pizza	290	38	2 ½	9	11	3.5	15	560	4
sausage	⅓ pizza	360	33	2	16	17	8.0	40	900	1
Wendy's®										
Baked potatoes										
plain	1	270	61	4	7	0	0.0	0	25	7
sour cream & chives	1	320	63	4	8	4	2.0	10	50	7
Chicken nuggets	5	230	13	1	12	14	3.0	35	430	0
Chicken nuggets, spicy	5	230	14	1	10	15	3.5	35	690	1
Chicken sandwiches										
crispy chicken	1	350	38	2 ½	15	15	3.0	35	830	2
go wrap, grilled	1	260	25	1 ½	20	10	3.5	55	750	1
go wrap, homestyle	1	320	29	2	15	16	4.5	35	760	1
spicy chicken	1	460	54	3 ½	26	16	3.0	60	1330	3
ultimate chicken grill	1	370	42	3	34	7	1.5	90	1150	2
Chili	small	220	22	1	18	7	3.0	35	870	6
Frosty™ shake, chocolate fudge										
small	1	410	69	4 ½	8	11	7.0	35	190	1
large	1	540	94	6	11	13	8.0	40	270	1
Frosty™ shake, vanilla bean										
small	1	380	64	4	7	11	7.0	35	140	0
large	1	510	88	6	9	13	8.0	40	180	0
Hamburgers, w/ standard toppings										
¼ lb. single	1	550	43	3	30	28	12.0	95	1280	2
½ lb. double	1	770	43	3	50	43	19.0	160	1450	2
Baconator™, single	1	630	43	3	33	36	15.0	110	1250	1
Jr. bacon cheeseburger	1	350	28	2	17	19	8.0	55	660	2
Jr. cheeseburger	1	270	26	2	15	11	5.0	40	690	1
Jr. cheeseburger deluxe	1	300	28	2	15	14	6.0	45	700	2
Jr. hamburger	1	230	26	2	12	8	3.0	30	480	1
Natural-cut French fries	medium	420	54	3 ½	5	20	3.5	0	500	6
Salad dressings										
avocado ranch	1 pkt.	100	1	0	1	10	2.0	10	220	0
creamy red jalapeño	1 pkt.	100	2	0	1	10	2.0	10	270	0
lemon garlic Caesar	1 pkt.	110	2	0	2	11	2.0	10	180	0
pomegranate vinaigrette	1 pkt.	60	8	½	0	3	0.0	0	160	0
Salads, w/o dressing										
apple pecan chicken	1	350	29	2	37	12	7.0	110	1210	5

FAST FOODS & RESTAURANT CHAINS

Wendys®

ITEM	AMOUNT	CALORIES	CARBOHYDRATE (g)	CARBOHYDRATE CHOICES	PROTEIN (g)	FAT (g)	SATURATED FAT (g)	CHOLESTEROL (mg)	SODIUM (mg)	FIBER (g)
Salads, w/o dressing *(continued)*										
Baja	1	550	36	2	33	33	14.0	85	1610	12
BLT cobb	1	460	12	1	46	26	12.0	285	1490	3
spicy chicken Caesar	1	450	25	1 ½	32	25	11.0	100	1290	6

FATS, OILS, CREAM & GRAVY

ITEM	AMOUNT	CALORIES	CARBOHYDRATE (g)	CARBOHYDRATE CHOICES	PROTEIN (g)	FAT (g)	SATURATED FAT (g)	CHOLESTEROL (mg)	SODIUM (mg)	FIBER (g)
Bacon fat	1 T.	116	0	0	0	13	5.0	12	19	0
Beef fat/tallow	1 T.	108	0	0	0	12	6.0	13	0	0
Benecol® spread										
light	1 T.	50	0	0	0	5	0.5	0	110	0
regular	1 T.	70	0	0	0	8	1.0	0	110	0
Butter										
butter oil	1 T.	112	0	0	0	13	8.0	33	0	0
stick	1 tsp.	34	0	0	0	4	2.5	10	27	0
stick	1 T.	100	0	0	0	11	7.0	30	81	0
stick, unsalted	1 tsp.	34	0	0	0	4	2.5	10	1	0
whipped	1 tsp.	23	0	0	0	3	1.5	7	26	0
whipped, light	1 tsp.	15	0	0	0	2	1.0	5	27	0
Butter flavored sprinkles	1 tsp.	5	2	0	0	0	0.0	0	120	0
Chicken fat	1 T.	115	0	0	0	13	4.0	11	0	0
Coconut milk creamer	1 T.	10	1	0	0	0	0.0	0	0	0
Coffee-Mate®, liquid										
fat free	1 T.	10	1	0	0	0	0.0	0	0	0
fat free, flavored	1 T.	25	5	0	0	0	0.0	0	25	0
regular	1 T.	20	2	0	0	1	0.0	0	0	0
regular, flavored	1 T.	35	5	0	0	2	0.0	0	30	0
sugar free, flavored	1 T.	15	2	0	0	1	0.0	0	0	0
Coffee-Mate®, powder										
fat free	1 tsp.	10	2	0	0	0	0.0	0	0	0
fat free, flavored	1 T.	38	8	½	0	0	0.0	0	11	0
regular	1 tsp.	10	1	0	0	1	0.5	0	0	0
regular, flavored	1 T.	45	7	½	0	2	1.5	0	11	0
sugar free, flavored	1 T.	30	2	0	0	3	2.0	0	15	0
Coffee Rich®	1 T.	20	2	0	0	3	2.0	0	15	0
Cooking spray	⅓ second	0	0	0	0	0	0.0	0	0	0
Cooking spray	2 seconds	14	0	0	0	2	0.0	0	0	0
Cream										
heavy	1 T.	51	0	0	0	6	3.5	20	6	0
light	1 T.	29	1	0	0	3	2.0	10	6	0
Gravy, beef										
au jus, jar	¼ cup	20	2	0	1	1	0.0	0	340	0
brown, mix	¼ cup	20	3	0	1	1	0.0	0	380	0

FATS, OILS, CREAM & GRAVY

ITEM	AMOUNT	CALORIES	CARBOHYDRATE (g)	CARBOHYDRATE CHOICES	PROTEIN (g)	FAT (g)	SATURATED FAT (g)	CHOLESTEROL (mg)	SODIUM (mg)	FIBER (g)
Gravy, beef *(continued)*										
fat free, can	¼ cup	15	3	0	1	0	0.0	0	300	0
hmde.	¼ cup	53	4	0	1	4	1.0	1	390	0
regular, can	¼ cup	31	3	0	2	1	0.5	2	326	0
Gravy, chicken										
fat free, can	¼ cup	15	3	0	1	0	0.0	5	310	0
giblet, hmde.	¼ cup	49	3	0	3	3	0.5	28	341	0
mix	¼ cup	25	4	0	1	1	0.0	0	340	0
regular, can	¼ cup	47	3	0	1	3	1.0	1	343	0
Gravy, other										
mushroom, can	¼ cup	30	3	0	1	2	0.0	0	339	0
onion, mix	¼ cup	20	4	0	1	1	0.5	0	300	0
pork, can	¼ cup	25	4	0	1	0	0.0	0	230	0
sausage, can	¼ cup	70	6	½	1	5	1.5	5	270	0
turkey, can	¼ cup	30	3	0	2	1	0.5	1	344	0
turkey, mix	¼ cup	25	4	0	1	1	0.0	0	370	0
Half & half										
fat free	1 T.	10	2	0	1	0	0.0	0	13	0
regular	1 T.	20	1	0	0	2	1.0	6	6	0
Lard/pork fat	1 T.	116	0	0	0	13	5.0	12	0	0
Margarine										
fat free	1 tsp.	2	0	0	0	0	0.0	0	30	0
fat free	1 T.	5	0	0	0	0	0.0	0	90	0
light	1 tsp.	10	0	0	0	2	0.5	0	28	0
light	1 T.	30	0	0	0	5	1.0	0	85	0
regular, soft/tub	1 tsp.	33	0	0	0	4	1.0	0	42	0
regular, soft/tub	1 T.	100	0	0	0	11	3.0	0	125	0
regular, soft/tub, unsalted	1 T.	100	0	0	0	11	2.0	0	0	0
regular, stick	1 tsp.	33	0	0	0	4	1.0	0	38	0
regular, stick	1 T.	100	0	0	0	11	2.0	0	115	0
regular, stick, unsalted	1 T.	100	0	0	0	11	2.0	0	0	0
Mayonnaise										
fat free	1 T.	10	2	0	0	0	0.0	2	140	0
imitation, soy	1 T.	35	1	0	0	4	0.5	0	115	0
light	1 T.	50	1	0	0	5	0.5	5	120	0
regular	1 T.	100	0	0	0	11	1.5	5	75	0
Miracle Whip®										
Free®	1 T.	15	3	0	0	0	0.0	0	125	0
light	1 T.	20	2	0	0	2	0.0	0	130	0
regular	1 T.	40	2	0	0	4	0.5	0	105	0
Mocha Mix®										
fat free	1 T.	10	1	0	0	0	0.0	0	5	0

FATS, OILS, CREAM & GRAVY

ITEM	AMOUNT	CALORIES	CARBOHYDRATE (g)	CARBOHYDRATE CHOICES	PROTEIN (g)	FAT (g)	SATURATED FAT (g)	CHOLESTEROL (mg)	SODIUM (mg)	FIBER (g)
Mocha Mix® *(continued)*										
regular	1 T.	20	2	0	0	2	0.0	0	10	0
Oils										
avocado	1 T.	124	0	0	0	14	1.5	0	0	0
canola	1 T.	124	0	0	0	14	1.0	0	0	0
chili, flavored	1 T.	130	0	0	0	14	3.0	0	0	0
coconut	1 T.	117	0	0	0	14	12.0	0	0	0
cod liver/fish	1 T.	123	0	0	0	14	3.0	78	0	0
corn	1 T.	120	0	0	0	14	1.5	0	0	0
cottonseed	1 T.	120	0	0	0	14	3.5	0	0	0
flaxseed/linseed	1 T.	120	0	0	0	14	1.5	0	0	0
grapeseed	1 T.	120	0	0	0	14	1.5	0	0	0
olive	1 T.	119	0	0	0	14	2.0	0	0	0
palm	1 T.	120	0	0	0	14	6.5	0	0	0
palm kernel	1 T.	117	0	0	0	14	11.0	0	0	0
peanut	1 T.	119	0	0	0	14	2.5	0	0	0
safflower	1 T.	120	0	0	0	14	1.0	0	0	0
sesame	1 T.	120	0	0	0	14	2.0	0	0	0
soybean	1 T.	120	0	0	0	14	2.0	0	0	0
sunflower	1 T.	120	0	0	0	14	1.5	0	0	0
walnut	1 T.	120	0	0	0	14	1.0	0	0	0
wheat germ	1 T.	120	0	0	0	14	2.5	0	0	0
Popcorn topping	1 T.	120	0	0	0	14	2.0	0	0	0
Shortening, vegetable	1 T.	110	0	0	0	12	3.0	0	0	0
Silk® creamer										
French vanilla	1 T.	20	3	0	0	1	0.0	0	10	0
original	1 T.	15	1	0	0	1	0.0	0	10	0
Sour cream										
fat free	1 T.	15	2	0	1	0	0.0	1	12	0
imitation, soy	1 T.	23	2	0	1	2	0.0	0	28	0
light	1 T.	20	1	0	1	1	1.0	5	10	0
regular	1 T.	31	1	0	1	3	2.0	6	8	0
Yogurt spread	1 T.	45	0	0	0	5	1.0	0	90	0

FISH & SEAFOOD
(Cooked w/o fat unless indicated.)

ITEM	AMOUNT	CALORIES	CARBOHYDRATE (g)	CARBOHYDRATE CHOICES	PROTEIN (g)	FAT (g)	SATURATED FAT (g)	CHOLESTEROL (mg)	SODIUM (mg)	FIBER (g)
Abalone										
baked/broiled	3 oz.	119	7	½	19	1	0.0	96	341	0
flour fried	3 oz.	161	9	½	17	6	1.5	80	503	0
Anchovies, oil pack, can	3	25	0	0	4	1	0.5	10	440	0
Anchovy paste	1 tsp.	10	2	0	1	0	0.0	3	624	0

FISH & SEAFOOD

ITEM	AMOUNT	CALORIES	CARBOHYDRATE (g)	CARBOHYDRATE CHOICES	PROTEIN (g)	FAT (g)	SATURATED FAT (g)	CHOLESTEROL (mg)	SODIUM (mg)	FIBER (g)
Bass										
freshwater	3 oz.	124	0	0	21	4	1.0	74	77	0
sea/striped	3 oz.	106	0	0	19	3	0.5	88	75	0
Bluefish	3 oz.	135	0	0	22	5	1.0	65	66	0
Burbot	3 oz.	98	0	0	21	1	0.0	66	106	0
Butterfish	3 oz.	159	0	0	19	9	2.5	71	97	0
Calamari/squid										
baked/broiled	3 oz.	118	3	0	16	4	1.0	240	76	0
flour fried	3 oz.	149	7	½	15	6	1.5	221	260	0
Carp										
baked/broiled	3 oz.	138	0	0	19	6	1.0	71	54	0
flour fried	3 oz.	239	11	1	18	13	3.0	84	175	0
Catfish, farmed										
baked/broiled	3 oz.	129	0	0	16	7	1.5	54	68	0
flour fried	3 oz.	195	7	½	15	11	3.0	69	238	1
Catfish, wild	3 oz.	89	0	0	16	2	0.5	61	43	0
Caviar, black/red	1 T.	40	1	0	4	3	0.5	94	240	0
Cisco, smoked	3 oz.	151	0	0	14	10	1.5	27	409	0
Clams										
breaded & fried	10 small	190	10	½	13	11	2.5	57	342	0
raw	6 large	89	3	0	15	1	0.0	41	67	0
stuffed, frzn.	1 (2.2 oz.)	110	12	1	5	5	0.0	0	390	1
Cod, Atlantic/Pacific										
baked/broiled	3 oz.	89	0	0	19	1	0.0	47	66	0
breaded & fried	3 oz.	149	6	½	15	7	1.5	43	78	0
dried, salted	3 oz.	247	0	0	53	2	0.5	129	5976	0
Crab										
Alaska king	3 oz.	83	0	0	17	1	0.0	45	912	0
blue, can	½ cup	67	0	0	14	1	0.0	60	225	0
blue, fresh	3 oz.	87	0	0	17	2	0.0	85	237	0
dungeness	3 oz.	94	1	0	19	1	0.0	65	322	0
imitation	3 oz.	81	13	1	7	0	0.0	17	715	0
snow	3 oz.	117	0	0	16	5	1.0	80	270	0
soft shell, flour fried	3 oz.	284	15	1	17	17	3.5	105	283	1
Crab cakes	1 (2 oz.)	160	5	0	11	10	2.0	82	491	0
Crawdads/crayfish	3 oz.	70	0	0	14	1	0.0	113	80	0
Croaker, breaded & fried	3 oz.	188	6	½	16	11	3.0	71	296	0
Cusk	3 oz.	95	0	0	21	1	0.0	45	34	0
Cuttlefish	3 oz.	134	1	0	28	1	0.0	191	633	0
Dolphinfish/mahi mahi	3 oz.	93	0	0	20	1	0.0	80	96	0
Drum, freshwater	3 oz.	130	0	0	19	5	1.0	70	82	0
Eel	3 oz.	201	0	0	20	13	2.5	137	55	0

FISH & SEAFOOD

ITEM	AMOUNT	CALORIES	CARBOHYDRATE (g)	CARBOHYDRATE CHOICES	PROTEIN (g)	FAT (g)	SATURATED FAT (g)	CHOLESTEROL (mg)	SODIUM (mg)	FIBER (g)
Escargot/snails	6	82	5	0	14	0	0.0	39	105	0
Fish cakes, breaded, frzn.	1 (3 oz.)	231	15	1	8	15	6.0	22	152	1
Fish fillets, frzn.	1 (3.5 oz.)	230	16	1	11	14	3.5	30	400	0
Fish sticks, frzn.	6 (0.6 oz.)	260	19	1	10	16	4.0	25	340	1
Flounder										
baked/broiled	3 oz.	100	0	0	21	1	0.5	58	89	0
breaded & fried	3 oz.	189	7	½	17	10	2.0	59	157	0
Gefiltefish	3 oz.	71	6	½	8	2	0.5	26	446	0
Grouper	3 oz.	100	0	0	21	1	0.5	40	45	0
Haddock										
baked/broiled	3 oz.	95	0	0	21	1	0.0	63	74	0
breaded & fried	3 oz.	196	14	1	10	12	2.0	23	399	0
smoked	3 oz.	99	0	0	22	1	0.0	66	649	0
Halibut										
Atlantic/Pacific	3 oz.	119	0	0	23	3	0.5	35	59	0
Greenland	3 oz.	203	0	0	16	15	2.5	50	88	0
Herring, Atlantic										
baked/broiled	3 oz.	173	0	0	20	10	2.0	66	98	0
pickled	1 (0.7 oz.)	52	2	0	3	4	0.5	3	174	0
Herring, Pacific	3 oz.	213	0	0	18	15	3.5	84	81	0
Ling/lingcod	3 oz.	93	0	0	19	1	0.0	57	65	0
Lobster										
Northern, breaded & fried	3 oz.	180	7	½	16	9	2.0	66	300	0
Northern, broiled/steamed	3 oz.	83	1	0	17	1	0.0	61	323	0
spiny, steamed	3 oz.	122	3	0	23	2	0.5	77	193	0
Lox/smoked salmon	3 oz.	100	0	0	16	4	1.0	20	1701	0
Mackerel										
Atlantic	3 oz.	223	0	0	20	15	3.5	64	71	0
Jack/Pacific	3 oz.	171	0	0	22	9	2.5	51	94	0
king	3 oz.	114	0	0	22	2	0.5	58	173	0
Spanish	3 oz.	134	0	0	20	5	1.5	62	56	0
Milkfish	3 oz.	162	0	0	22	7	2.0	57	78	0
Mollusks/whelk	3 oz.	234	13	1	41	1	0.0	111	350	0
Monkfish	3 oz.	83	0	0	16	2	0.5	27	20	0
Mullet, striped	3 oz.	128	0	0	21	4	1.0	54	60	0
Mussels	3 oz.	146	6	½	20	4	0.5	48	314	0
Octopus	3 oz.	140	4	0	25	2	0.5	82	391	0
Orange roughy	3 oz.	76	0	0	19	1	0.0	68	59	0
Oysters										
Eastern, breaded & fried	6 (0.5 oz.)	173	10	½	8	11	3.0	71	367	0
Eastern, raw	6 (0.5 oz.)	50	5	0	4	1	0.5	21	150	0
Pacific, raw	3 (1.8 oz.)	122	7	½	14	3	1.0	75	159	0

FISH & SEAFOOD

ITEM	AMOUNT	CALORIES	CARBOHYDRATE (g)	CARBOHYDRATE CHOICES	PROTEIN (g)	FAT (g)	SATURATED FAT (g)	CHOLESTEROL (mg)	SODIUM (mg)	FIBER (g)
Oysters *(continued)*										
smoked, oil pack, can	3 oz.	150	9	½	15	9	3.0	60	315	0
Perch										
baked/broiled	3 oz.	103	0	0	20	2	0.5	46	82	0
breaded & fried	3 oz.	226	14	1	9	15	2.0	19	361	0
Pollock, Atlantic	3 oz.	96	0	0	20	1	0.0	82	99	0
Pompano, Florida	3 oz.	179	0	0	20	10	4.0	54	65	0
Pout	3 oz.	87	0	0	18	1	0.5	57	66	0
Rockfish, Pacific	3 oz.	103	0	0	20	2	0.5	37	66	0
Roe	3 oz.	174	2	0	24	7	1.5	407	100	0
Sablefish	3 oz.	213	0	0	15	17	3.5	54	61	0
Salmon										
Atlantic	3 oz.	155	0	0	22	7	1.0	60	48	0
Chinook	3 oz.	197	0	0	22	11	2.5	72	51	0
coho	3 oz.	151	0	0	21	7	1.5	54	44	0
pink, can	3 oz.	122	0	0	16	7	1.5	54	365	0
sockeye, can	3 oz.	141	0	0	20	6	1.5	37	306	0
Sardines, oil pack, can	2	50	0	0	6	3	0.5	34	121	0
Scallops										
bay, baked/broiled	3 oz.	142	5	0	27	1	0.0	61	314	0
imitation	3 oz.	84	9	½	11	0	0.0	19	676	0
sea, baked/broiled	6 large	140	5	0	27	1	0.0	60	310	0
sea, breaded & fried	6 large	200	9	½	17	10	2.5	57	432	0
Scup	3 oz.	115	0	0	21	3	1.0	57	46	0
Shad	3 oz.	214	0	0	18	15	4.0	82	55	0
Shad roe	½ cup	183	2	0	24	10	2.5	400	139	0
Shark	3 oz.	153	0	0	21	7	1.5	51	108	0
Shrimp										
baked/broiled/raw	10 large	55	0	0	12	1	0.0	107	123	0
breaded & fried	10 large	182	9	½	16	9	1.5	133	258	0
Smelt, rainbow										
baked/broiled	3 oz.	106	0	0	19	3	0.5	77	66	0
flour fried	3 oz.	217	11	1	18	11	2.5	88	188	0
Snapper	3 oz.	109	0	0	22	2	0.5	40	49	0
Sole										
baked/broiled	3 oz.	100	0	0	21	1	0.5	58	89	0
breaded & fried	3 oz.	189	7	½	17	10	2.0	59	157	0
Sturgeon										
baked/broiled	3 oz.	115	0	0	18	4	1.0	66	59	0
flour fried	3 oz.	199	7	½	15	12	2.5	68	133	0
smoked	3 oz.	147	0	0	27	4	1.0	68	629	0
Sucker, white	3 oz.	101	0	0	18	3	0.5	45	43	0

FISH & SEAFOOD

ITEM	AMOUNT	CALORIES	CARBOHYDRATE (g)	CARBOHYDRATE CHOICES	PROTEIN (g)	FAT (g)	SATURATED FAT (g)	CHOLESTEROL (mg)	SODIUM (mg)	FIBER (g)
Sunfish	3 oz.	97	0	0	21	1	0.0	73	88	0
Swordfish	3 oz.	132	0	0	22	4	1.0	43	98	0
Tilefish	3 oz.	125	0	0	21	4	0.5	54	50	0
Trout, rainbow										
baked/broiled	3 oz.	128	0	0	19	5	1.5	59	48	0
flour fried	3 oz.	230	9	½	20	13	2.5	72	151	0
Tuna, can										
light, oil pack	¼ cup	110	0	0	13	6	1.0	30	250	0
light, water pack	¼ cup	60	0	0	13	1	0.0	30	250	0
low sodium, water pack	¼ cup	70	0	0	15	1	0.0	25	35	0
white, oil pack	¼ cup	90	0	0	13	4	1.0	25	210	0
white, water pack	¼ cup	70	0	0	15	1	0.0	25	250	0
Tuna, fresh										
bluefin	3 oz.	156	0	0	25	5	1.5	42	43	0
yellowfin	3 oz.	118	0	0	26	1	0.5	49	40	0
Turbot	3 oz.	104	0	0	18	3	0.5	53	163	0
Walleye	3 oz.	101	0	0	21	1	0.5	94	55	0
Whitefish	3 oz.	146	0	0	21	6	1.0	66	55	0
Whiting	3 oz.	99	0	0	20	1	0.5	71	112	0
Wolffish, Atlantic	3 oz.	105	0	0	19	3	0.5	50	93	0
Yellowtail	3 oz.	159	0	0	25	6	1.0	60	43	0

FRUIT & VEGETABLE JUICES
Fruit Juices & Nectars

ITEM	AMOUNT	CALORIES	CARBOHYDRATE (g)	CARBOHYDRATE CHOICES	PROTEIN (g)	FAT (g)	SATURATED FAT (g)	CHOLESTEROL (mg)	SODIUM (mg)	FIBER (g)
Apple-cherry	1 cup	117	29	2	1	0	0.0	0	6	1
Apple cider/juice	1 cup	117	29	2	0	0	0.0	0	7	0
Apricot nectar	1 cup	141	36	2 ½	1	0	0.0	0	8	2
Cranberry cocktail										
red, light	1 cup	40	10	½	0	0	0.0	0	75	0
red, regular	1 cup	130	33	2	0	0	0.0	0	35	0
white, regular	1 cup	120	29	2	0	0	0.0	0	35	0
Cran-Apple®	1 cup	130	32	2	0	0	0.0	0	80	
Cran-Peach	1 cup	110	27	2	0	0	0.0	0	50	0
Cran-Pomegranate™	1 cup	120	30	2	0	0	0.0	0	35	0
Cran-Raspberry®										
light	1 cup	40	10	½	0	0	0.0	0	70	0
regular	1 cup	110	28	2	0	0	0.0	0	70	0
Grape										
purple, light	1 cup	70	18	1	0	0	0.0	0	70	0
purple, regular	1 cup	170	42	3	0	0	0.0	0	20	0
white, regular	1 cup	160	39	2 ½	0	0	0.0	0	20	0
white, sparkling, regular	1 cup	160	40	2 ½	0	0	0.0	0	45	0

FRUIT & VEGETABLE JUICES

Fruit Juices & Nectars

ITEM	AMOUNT	CALORIES	CARBOHYDRATE (g)	CARBOHYDRATE CHOICES	PROTEIN (g)	FAT (g)	SATURATED FAT (g)	CHOLESTEROL (mg)	SODIUM (mg)	FIBER (g)
Grapefruit										
red, light	1 cup	40	10	½	0	0	0.0	0	65	0
red, regular	1 cup	130	32	2	0	0	0.0	0	35	0
white, regular	1 cup	90	21	1 ½	2	0	0.0	0	35	0
Guava nectar	1 cup	149	38	2 ½	0	0	0.0	0	7	2
Lemon	2 T.	8	3	0	0	0	0.0	0	0	0
Lime	2 T.	8	3	0	0	0	0.0	0	0	0
Mango	1 cup	140	34	2	0	1	0.0	0	70	0
Orange	1 cup	110	27	2	1	0	0.0	0	15	0
Peach juice/nectar	1 cup	135	35	2	1	0	0.0	0	17	2
Pear juice/nectar	1 cup	150	39	2 ½	0	0	0.0	0	10	2
Pineapple, unsweetened	1 cup	133	32	2	1	0	0.0	0	5	1
Pomegranate										
light	1 cup	40	9	½	0	0	0.0	0	10	0
regular	1 cup	140	34	2	0	0	0.0	0	15	0
Prune	1 cup	182	45	3	2	0	0.0	0	10	3
Twister®										
blue raspberry rush	1 cup	110	26	2	0	0	0.0	0	25	0
orange strawberry banana burst	1 cup	130	33	2	0	0	0.0	0	25	0
strawberry kiwi cyclone	1 cup	120	30	2	0	0	0.0	0	25	0
tropical fruit fury	1 cup	140	35	2	0	0	0.0	0	25	0
Vegetable Juices										
Carrot	1 cup	94	22	1 ½	2	0	0.0	0	68	2
Clamato®	1 cup	50	11	1	1	0	0.0	0	870	1
Tomato	1 cup	50	10	½	2	0	0.0	0	680	1
V-8®										
low sodium	1 cup	50	10	½	2	0	0.0	0	140	2
regular	1 cup	50	10	½	2	0	0.0	0	420	2
V-8® Fusion™										
peach mango	1 cup	120	28	2	1	0	0.0	0	70	0
pomegranate blueberry	1 cup	100	25	1 ½	0	0	0.0	0	60	0
V-8® Splash®										
tropical blend, diet	1 cup	10	3	0	0	0	0.0	0	30	0
tropical blend, regular	1 cup	70	18	1	0	0	0.0	0	50	0
tropical colada	1 cup	100	21	1 ½	3	0	0.0	0	50	1

FRUITS

ITEM	AMOUNT	CALORIES	CARBOHYDRATE (g)	CARBOHYDRATE CHOICES	PROTEIN (g)	FAT (g)	SATURATED FAT (g)	CHOLESTEROL (mg)	SODIUM (mg)	FIBER (g)
Apples										
dried	4 rings	62	17	1	0	0	0.0	0	22	2
fresh	1 medium	80	22	1	0	1	0.0	0	0	5

FRUITS

ITEM	AMOUNT	CALORIES	CARBOHYDRATE (g)	CARBOHYDRATE CHOICES	PROTEIN (g)	FAT (g)	SATURATED FAT (g)	CHOLESTEROL (mg)	SODIUM (mg)	FIBER (g)
Applesauce										
natural/unsweetened	½ cup	53	14	1	0	0	0.0	0	2	2
sweetened	½ cup	97	25	1 ½	0	0	0.0	0	36	2
Apricots										
dried	4 medium	80	19	1	1	0	0.0	0	0	3
fresh	1 medium	17	4	0	1	0	0.0	0	0	1
heavy syrup, can	½ cup	107	28	2	1	0	0.0	0	5	2
light syrup, can	½ cup	80	21	1 ½	1	0	0.0	0	5	2
Avocados	½ medium	161	9	0	2	15	2.0	0	7	7
Banana chips	¼ cup	150	9	½	1	7	6.0	0	0	0
Bananas, fresh	1 medium	105	27	2	1	0	0.0	0	1	3
Blackberries, fresh	1 cup	62	14	½	2	1	0.0	0	1	7
Blueberries, fresh/frzn.	1 cup	84	21	1 ½	1	1	0.0	0	2	4
Boysenberries, fresh	1 cup	62	14	½	2	1	0.0	0	1	7
Breadfruit, fresh	¼ medium	99	26	1 ½	1	0	0.0	0	2	5
Cantaloupe, fresh	1 cup	54	13	1	1	0	0.0	0	26	1
Casaba melon, fresh	1 cup	48	11	1	2	0	0.0	0	15	2
Cherries, red										
maraschino	1 medium	10	3	0	0	0	0.0	0	0	0
sour, fresh	½ cup	39	9	½	1	0	0.0	0	2	1
sour, heavy syrup, can	½ cup	117	30	2	1	0	0.0	0	9	1
sweet, fresh	12 medium	51	13	1	1	1	0.0	0	0	2
sweet, heavy syrup, can	½ cup	105	27	2	1	0	0.0	0	4	2
Coconut, shredded										
fresh	¼ cup	71	3	0	1	7	6.0	0	4	2
sweetened, dried	¼ cup	117	11	1	1	8	7.5	0	61	1
Cranberries										
Craisins®/sweetened, dried	⅓ cup	130	33	2	0	0	0.0	0	0	3
fresh/frzn.	½ cup	22	6	½	0	0	0.0	0	1	2
Currants, fresh	½ cup	35	9	½	1	0	0.0	0	1	4
Dates, dried	¼ cup	126	33	2	1	0	0.0	0	1	4
Figs										
dried	2 medium	95	24	1 ½	1	0	0.0	0	4	4
fresh	2 medium	74	19	1	1	0	0.0	0	1	3
Fruit cocktail										
heavy syrup, can	½ cup	91	23	1 ½	1	0	0.0	0	7	1
light syrup, can	½ cup	69	18	1	1	0	0.0	0	7	1
Gooseberries, fresh	1 cup	66	15	11	1	0	0.0	2	7	
Grapefruit										
light syrup, can	½ cup	76	20	1	1	0	0.0	0	3	1
sections, fresh	1 cup	74	19	1	1	0	0.0	0	0	3
whole, fresh	½ medium	39	10	½	1	0	0.0	0	0	1

FRUITS

ITEM	AMOUNT	CALORIES	CARBOHYDRATE (g)	CARBOHYDRATE CHOICES	PROTEIN (g)	FAT (g)	SATURATED FAT (g)	CHOLESTEROL (mg)	SODIUM (mg)	FIBER (g)
Grapes, fresh	15 medium	52	14	1	1	0	0.0	0	2	1
Guavas, fresh	1 medium	61	13	½	2	1	0.0	0	2	5
Honeydew melon, fresh	1 cup	61	16	1	1	0	0.0	0	31	1
Kiwifruit, fresh	1 medium	46	11	1	1	0	0.0	0	4	3
Kumquats, fresh	1 medium	14	3	0	0	0	0.0	0	2	1
Lemons, fresh	½ medium	8	3	0	0	0	0.0	0	1	1
Limes, fresh	½ medium	10	4	0	0	0	0.0	0	1	1
Loganberries, fresh	1 cup	62	14	½	2	1	0.0	0	1	7
Mandarin oranges, can	½ cup	46	12	1	1	0	0.0	0	6	1
Mangoes, fresh	½ medium	67	18	1	1	0	0.0	0	2	2
Melon balls, frzn.	1 cup	57	14	1	2	0	0.0	0	54	1
Mixed fruit										
dried	¼ cup	120	28	2	1	0	0.0	0	55	2
sweetened, frzn.	½ cup	123	30	2	2	0	0.0	0	4	2
Mulberries, fresh	1 cup	60	14	1	2	1	0.0	0	14	2
Nectarines, fresh	1 medium	63	15	1	2	1	0.0	0	0	2
Oranges, fresh	1 medium	62	15	1	1	0	0.0	0	0	3
Papayas, fresh	½ medium	59	15	1	1	0	0.0	0	5	3
Passion fruit, fresh	1 medium	18	4	0	0	0	0.0	0	5	2
Peaches										
fresh	1 medium	39	9	½	1	0	0.0	0	0	2
heavy syrup, can	½ cup	97	26	2	1	0	0.0	0	8	2
light syrup, can	½ cup	68	18	1	1	0	0.0	0	6	2
Pears										
fresh	1 medium	96	26	1 ½	1	0	0.0	0	2	5
heavy syrup, can	½ cup	98	26	2	0	0	0.0	0	7	2
light syrup, can	½ cup	72	19	1	0	0	0.0	0	6	2
Persimmons, native, fresh	1 medium	32	8	½	0	0	0.0	0	0	0
Pineapple chunks										
fresh	1 cup	74	20	1	1	0	0.0	0	2	2
heavy syrup, can	½ cup	99	26	2	0	0	0.0	0	1	1
light syrup, can	½ cup	66	17	1	1	0	0.0	0	1	1
Plantains, cooked	1 cup	179	48	3	1	0	0.0	0	8	4
Plums, fresh	1 medium	30	8	½	1	0	0.0	0	0	1
Pomegranates, fresh	½ medium	52	13	1	1	0	0.0	0	2	1
Prickly pears, fresh	1 medium	42	10	½	1	1	0.0	0	5	4
Prunes, dried	3 medium	61	16	1	1	0	0.0	0	1	2
Quince, fresh	1 medium	52	14	1	0	0	0.0	0	4	2
Raisins	¼ cup	123	33	2	1	0	0.0	0	5	2
Raspberries, fresh	1 cup	64	15	1	2	1	0.0	0	1	8
Rhubarb										
fresh	1 cup	26	6	½	1	0	0.0	0	5	2

FRUITS

ITEM	AMOUNT	CALORIES	CARBOHYDRATE (g)	CARBOHYDRATE CHOICES	PROTEIN (g)	FAT (g)	SATURATED FAT (g)	CHOLESTEROL (mg)	SODIUM (mg)	FIBER (g)
Rhubarb *(continued)*										
sweetened, cooked	½ cup	139	37	2 ½	1	0	0.0	0	1	2
Starfruit, fresh	1 medium	39	9	½	1	0	0.0	0	3	4
Strawberries										
fresh	1 cup	53	13	1	1	1	0.0	0	2	3
sweetened, frzn.	½ cup	122	33	2	1	0	0.0	0	4	2
Tangerines, fresh	1 medium	45	11	1	1	0	0.0	0	2	2
Tropical fruit, light, can	½ cup	80	21	1 ½	0	0	0.0	0	10	1
Watermelon, fresh	1 cup	46	12	1	1	0	0.0	0	2	1

MEATS

(Cooked w/o fat unless indicated.)

Beef

ITEM	AMOUNT	CALORIES	CARBOHYDRATE (g)	CARBOHYDRATE CHOICES	PROTEIN (g)	FAT (g)	SATURATED FAT (g)	CHOLESTEROL (mg)	SODIUM (mg)	FIBER (g)
Bottom round	3 oz.	190	0	0	28	8	2.5	104	37	0
Chuck roast										
arm	3 oz.	174	0	0	29	5	2.0	52	49	0
blade	3 oz.	214	0	0	26	11	4.5	90	60	0
Corned brisket	3 oz.	214	0	0	16	16	5.5	83	964	0
Eye of round	3 oz.	177	0	0	24	8	3.0	53	32	0
Filet mignon	3 oz.	185	0	0	24	10	3.5	71	48	0
Flank steak	3 oz.	165	0	0	24	7	3.0	47	48	0
Ground hamburger										
extra lean, 5% fat	3 oz.	145	0	0	22	6	2.5	65	55	0
lean, 10% fat	3 oz.	185	0	0	22	10	4.0	72	58	0
lean, 15% fat	3 oz.	213	0	0	22	13	5.0	77	61	0
regular, 20% fat	3 oz.	231	0	0	22	15	5.5	77	64	0
Ground round, extra lean	3 oz.	130	0	0	24	4	1.5	60	65	0
London broil	3 oz.	165	0	0	24	7	3.0	47	48	0
Porterhouse steak	3 oz.	173	0	0	23	8	3.5	49	59	0
Pot roast, chuck	3 oz.	253	0	0	25	16	6.5	81	40	0
Prime rib	3 oz.	350	0	0	19	30	12.5	71	55	0
Rib eye steak	3 oz.	196	0	0	24	11	4.0	82	50	0
Round steak	3 oz.	162	0	0	23	7	2.5	66	49	0
Rump roast	3 oz.	204	0	0	28	8	3.5	61	37	0
Short ribs	3 oz.	251	0	0	26	15	6.5	79	49	0
Sirloin steak	3 oz.	180	0	0	25	8	3.0	62	52	0
Sirloin tips	3 oz.	156	0	0	26	5	2.0	49	54	0
Stew meat	3 oz.	200	0	0	23	11	4.0	72	87	0
Strip steak	3 oz.	164	0	0	25	7	2.5	49	50	0
T-bone steak	3 oz.	174	0	0	23	9	3.0	50	66	0
Tenderloin, lean	3 oz.	164	0	0	24	7	2.5	67	50	0
Top round	3 oz.	158	0	0	27	5	2.0	56	35	0

MEATS
Beef

ITEM	AMOUNT	CALORIES	CARBOHYDRATE (g)	CARBOHYDRATE CHOICES	PROTEIN (g)	FAT (g)	SATURATED FAT (g)	CHOLESTEROL (mg)	SODIUM (mg)	FIBER (g)
Top sirloin	3 oz.	180	0	0	25	8	3.0	62	52	0
Veal										
chops	3 oz.	192	0	0	29	8	2.0	106	71	0
chops, breaded & fried	3 oz.	194	8	½	23	8	2.5	95	386	0
cutlets/loin chops, braised	3 oz.	242	0	0	26	15	5.5	100	68	0
ground	3 oz.	146	0	0	21	6	2.5	88	71	0
loin	3 oz.	149	0	0	22	6	2.0	90	82	0
patties, breaded & fried	3 oz.	208	11	1	10	14	6.0	34	243	1
shoulder	3 oz.	194	0	0	27	9	3.0	107	81	0
sirloin	3 oz.	143	0	0	22	5	2.0	88	72	0
Game										
Beefalo	3 oz.	160	0	0	26	5	2.5	49	70	0
Bison/buffalo	3 oz.	122	0	0	24	2	1.0	70	49	0
Rabbit										
domestic	3 oz.	168	0	0	25	7	2.0	70	40	0
wild	3 oz.	147	0	0	28	3	1.0	105	38	0
Venison	3 oz.	134	0	0	26	3	1.0	95	46	0
Lamb										
Chops	3 oz.	184	0	0	26	8	3.0	81	71	0
Leg	3 oz.	219	0	0	22	14	6.0	79	56	0
Shoulder	3 oz.	235	0	0	19	17	7.0	78	56	0
Pork										
Chops										
broiled	3 oz.	179	0	0	24	8	3.0	67	54	0
fried	3 oz.	219	0	0	25	13	4.5	66	47	0
Ground	3 oz.	253	0	0	22	18	6.5	80	62	0
Ham										
cured, lean	3 oz.	134	0	0	21	5	1.5	47	1129	0
hocks	3 oz.	280	0	0	24	20	7.0	93	75	0
leg, fresh	3 oz.	232	0	0	23	15	5.5	80	51	0
picnic/shoulder roast	3 oz.	194	0	0	23	11	3.5	81	68	0
Loin	3 oz.	203	0	0	23	12	4.5	68	41	0
Spareribs, lean	3 oz.	199	0	0	22	12	4.0	73	54	0
Tenderloin, lean	3 oz.	140	0	0	24	4	1.5	67	48	0
Processed & Luncheon Meats										
Bacon	1 slice	34	0	0	2	3	1.0	7	146	0
Bacon bits										
imitation	1 T.	20	1	0	2	1	0.0	0	147	0

MEATS
Processed & Luncheon Meats

ITEM	AMOUNT	CALORIES	CARBOHYDRATE (g)	CARBOHYDRATE CHOICES	PROTEIN (g)	FAT (g)	SATURATED FAT (g)	CHOLESTEROL (mg)	SODIUM (mg)	FIBER (g)
Bacon bits *(continued)*										
real	1 T.	25	0	0	3	2	1.0	5	240	0
Beef jerky	1 oz.	80	5	0	13	1	0.0	25	650	0
Beef sticks/Slim Jim®	1 (8.5 inch)	90	1	0	4	8	3.0	10	280	0
Bologna										
beef/beef & pork	1 oz.	90	1	0	3	8	3.5	20	310	0
turkey, fat free	1 oz.	25	3	0	3	1	0.0	10	240	0
Braunschweiger	1 oz.	93	1	0	4	8	2.5	51	329	0
Canadian bacon	1 oz.	45	1	0	6	2	0.5	14	399	0
Corned beef, can	2 oz.	120	0	0	14	7	3.0	40	490	0
Corned beef hash, can	1 cup	390	22	1 ½	21	24	11.0	80	1000	2
Deviled ham® spread	¼ cup	180	1	0	8	15	5.0	35	480	0
Ham, chopped, can	2 oz.	90	0	0	9	6	2.0	30	620	0
Ham, deli, extra-lean	1 oz.	31	1	0	5	1	0.5	14	314	0
Headcheese	1 oz.	76	0	0	4	6	2.0	16	189	0
Hot dogs										
beef	1 (1.6 oz.)	130	1	0	5	12	5.0	30	470	0
beef, bun length	1 (2 oz.)	170	1	0	7	15	7.0	40	590	0
beef, w/ cheese	1 (1.6 oz.)	140	1	0	5	13	4.0	35	540	0
chicken/pork/turkey	1 (1.6 oz.)	130	1	0	5	12	4.0	35	540	0
Liverwurst	1 oz.	92	1	0	4	8	3.0	45	244	0
Mortadella	1 oz.	88	1	0	5	7	2.5	16	353	0
Olive loaf	1 oz.	75	2	0	3	6	2.0	20	374	0
Pastrami	1 oz.	45	1	0	7	2	0.5	17	249	0
Pepperoni	1 oz.	130	0	0	6	12	4.5	25	470	0
Roast beef, deli	1 oz.	32	0	0	6	1	0.5	14	287	0
Salami										
beef	1 oz.	74	1	0	4	6	3.0	20	323	0
beef & pork/Genoa	1 oz.	110	0	0	6	9	3.5	29	518	0
Sandwich steaks, frzn.	1 (2 oz.)	175	0	0	9	15	6.5	40	39	0
Sausages										
bockwurst	1 (2 oz.)	158	0	0	6	15	6.0	53	282	0
bratwurst	1 (2 oz.)	189	2	0	8	17	5.5	42	480	0
breakfast	1 (0.7 oz.)	80	1	0	2	7	2.5	15	140	0
chorizo	1 (2 oz.)	258	1	0	14	22	8.0	50	700	0
Italian	1 (2 oz.)	195	2	0	11	16	5.5	32	684	0
kielbasa	1 (2 oz.)	176	1	0	8	15	5.5	38	610	0
knockwurst	1 (2 oz.)	174	2	0	6	16	6.0	34	527	0
Polish	1 (2 oz.)	185	1	0	8	16	6.0	40	497	0
smoked, beef	1 (2 oz.)	177	1	0	8	15	5.5	38	641	0
smoked, pork	1 (2 oz.)	221	1	0	13	18	6.5	39	851	0
summer	1 (1 oz.)	88	1	0	4	8	3.5	23	404	0

MEATS

Processed & Luncheon Meats

ITEM	AMOUNT	CALORIES	CARBOHYDRATE (g)	CARBOHYDRATE CHOICES	PROTEIN (g)	FAT (g)	SATURATED FAT (g)	CHOLESTEROL (mg)	SODIUM (mg)	FIBER (g)
Sausages *(continued)*										
Vienna	1 (0.6 oz.)	43	0	0	2	4	1.5	13	87	0
Spam®, can										
lite	2 oz.	110	1	0	9	8	3.0	40	580	0
reduced sodium	2 oz.	180	1	0	7	16	6.0	40	580	0
regular	2 oz.	180	1	0	7	16	6.0	40	790	0
Specialty & Organ Meats										
Brains, beef, pan fried	3 oz.	167	0	0	11	14	3.0	1697	134	0
Chitterlings, pork	3 oz.	198	0	0	11	17	8.0	236	15	0
Frog legs	3 oz.	90	0	0	20	0	0.0	62	72	0
Hearts, beef	3 oz.	140	0	0	24	4	1.0	180	50	0
Liver, beef, pan fried	3 oz.	149	4	0	23	4	1.5	324	66	0
Oxtail, beef, salted	3 oz.	207	0	0	26	11	5.0	94	162	0
Pigs' feet, pickled	3 oz.	119	0	0	10	9	2.5	71	476	0
Sweetbreads	1 oz.	66	0	0	7	4	2.0	113	15	0
Tongue, beef	3 oz.	242	0	0	16	19	7.0	112	55	0
Tripe, beef	3 oz.	80	2	0	10	3	1.0	134	58	0

MILK & YOGURT

Milk & Milk Beverages

ITEM	AMOUNT	CALORIES	CARBOHYDRATE (g)	CARBOHYDRATE CHOICES	PROTEIN (g)	FAT (g)	SATURATED FAT (g)	CHOLESTEROL (mg)	SODIUM (mg)	FIBER (g)
Acidophilus milk										
lowfat	1 cup	110	13	1	9	3	1.5	15	130	0
skim	1 cup	100	14	1	10	0	0.0	6	140	0
Almond milk										
regular	1 cup	60	8	½	1	3	0.0	0	150	1
unsweetened	1 cup	35	1	0	1	3	0.0	0	150	1
Buttermilk										
dried	1 T.	29	4	0	3	0	0.0	5	39	0
lowfat	1 cup	100	13	1	8	2	1.0	10	340	0
skim	1 cup	90	13	1	9	0	0.0	0	220	0
Chocolate milk										
lowfat	1 cup	158	26	2	8	3	1.5	8	153	1
skim	1 cup	148	30	2	8	1	0.5	4	144	1
whole	1 cup	208	26	2	8	9	5.5	30	150	2
Coconut milk										
regular	1 cup	80	7	½	1	5	5.0	0	15	0
unsweetened	1 cup	50	1	0	1	5	5.0	0	15	0
Coconut milk, can										
lite	¼ cup	48	2	0	1	4	3.0	0	15	0
regular	¼ cup	93	2	0	2	9	9.0	0	9	0

MILK & YOGURT
Milk & Milk Beverages

ITEM	AMOUNT	CALORIES	CARBOHYDRATE (g)	CARBOHYDRATE CHOICES	PROTEIN (g)	FAT (g)	SATURATED FAT (g)	CHOLESTEROL (mg)	SODIUM (mg)	FIBER (g)
Condensed milk, sweetened, can										
fat free	2 T.	110	24	1 ½	3	0	0.0	0	40	0
lowfat	2 T.	120	23	1 ½	3	2	1.0	5	40	0
whole	2 T.	130	23	1 ½	3	3	2.0	10	40	0
Eggnog, non-alcoholic										
lowfat	1 cup	140	23	1 ½	7	3	2.0	35	130	0
whole	1 cup	343	34	2	10	19	11.0	150	137	0
Evaporated milk, can										
lowfat	½ cup	100	12	1	8	2	2.0	20	140	0
skim	½ cup	100	15	1	10	0	0.0	5	147	0
whole	½ cup	169	13	1	9	10	6.0	37	134	0
Filled milk	1 cup	154	12	1	8	8	7.5	5	139	0
Goat milk	1 cup	168	11	1	9	10	6.5	27	122	0
Human breast milk	½ cup	86	9	½	1	5	2.5	17	21	0
Instant Breakfast®, dry										
chocolate, no added sugar	1 pkt.	60	12	1	5	1	0.0	0	60	4
chocolate, regular	1 pkt.	130	27	2	5	1	0.0	0	90	0
vanilla, regular	1 pkt.	130	27	2	5	0	0.0	0	100	0
Instant Breakfast®, prepared, w/ skim										
chocolate, no added sugar	1 cup	140	25	1 ½	13	1	0.0	5	185	4
chocolate, regular	1 cup	210	40	2 ½	13	1	0.0	5	205	0
vanilla, regular	1 cup	210	40	2 ½	13	0	0.0	5	225	0
Kefir										
flavored, lowfat	1 cup	174	25	1 ½	14	2	1.5	10	125	3
plain, lowfat	1 cup	120	12	1	14	2	1.5	10	125	3
plain, nonfat	1 cup	116	15	1	14	0	0.0	5	120	3
Lactaid® milk										
1%	1 cup	110	13	1	8	3	1.5	15	125	0
2%	1 cup	130	13	1	8	5	3.0	20	125	0
skim	1 cup	80	13	1	8	0	0.0	0	125	0
whole	1 cup	150	12	1	8	8	5.0	35	125	0
Lowfat milk										
1%	1 cup	110	12	1	8	3	1.5	15	125	0
1%, protein fortified	1 cup	118	14	1	10	3	2.0	10	143	0
2%	1 cup	130	13	1	8	5	3.0	20	125	0
Malted milk drink	1 cup	225	30	2	9	9	5.0	27	159	1
Milk shake, w/ whole										
chocolate	1 cup	211	34	2	6	6	4.0	22	161	3
vanilla	1 cup	246	33	2	6	11	6.5	38	135	2
Ovaltine®, w/ skim										
chocolate malt	1 cup	170	31	2	9	0	0.0	5	240	0
malt	1 cup	170	31	2	10	0	0.0	5	180	0

MILK & YOGURT
Milk & Milk Beverages

ITEM	AMOUNT	CALORIES	CARBOHYDRATE (g)	CARBOHYDRATE CHOICES	PROTEIN (g)	FAT (g)	SATURATED FAT (g)	CHOLESTEROL (mg)	SODIUM (mg)	FIBER (g)
Powdered milk, dry										
nonfat	¼ cup	61	9	½	6	0	0.0	3	93	0
whole	¼ cup	159	12	1	8	9	5.5	31	119	0
Rice Dream® rice drink										
plain	1 cup	120	23	1 ½	1	3	0.0	0	80	0
vanilla	1 cup	130	26	2	1	3	0.0	0	80	0
Sheep milk	1 cup	265	13	1	15	17	11.5	66	108	0
Silk® soy milk										
chocolate, light	1 cup	90	15	1	3	2	0.0	0	80	2
chocolate, regular	1 cup	140	23	1 ½	5	3	0.5	0	100	2
plain, light	1 cup	60	6	½	6	2	0.0	0	125	1
plain, regular	1 cup	100	8	½	6	4	0.5	0	120	1
plain, unsweetened	1 cup	80	4	0	7	4	0.5	0	85	1
vanilla, light	1 cup	70	7	½	6	2	0.0	0	100	1
vanilla, regular	1 cup	100	11	1	6	4	0.5	0	95	1
Skim milk	1 cup	80	13	1	8	0	0.0	5	125	0
Strawberry milk, Nesquik®, 1%	1 cup	180	31	2	8	5	3.0	15	10	0
Whole milk	1 cup	150	12	1	8	8	5.0	35	125	0
Yogurt										
Flavored										
fat free, w/ aspartame, fruited	1 (6 oz.)	100	19	1	5	0	0.0	0	85	0
light, fruited	1 cup	110	15	1	8	2	1.0	15	105	0
lowfat, fruited	1 cup	220	42	3	7	2	1.5	15	115	0
lowfat, w/ granola topping	1 (6 oz.)	190	38	2 ½	6	2	1.0	5	90	1
Greek										
nonfat, fruited	1 (6 oz.)	140	20	1	14	0	0.0	0	65	0
nonfat, plain	1 (6 oz.)	100	7	½	18	0	0.0	0	80	0
lowfat, fruited	1 (6 oz.)	160	19	1	14	3	2.0	5	65	1
lowfat, plain	1 (6 oz.)	130	7	½	17	4	2.0	10	70	0
Plain										
fat free	1 cup	110	16	1	11	0	0.0	5	150	0
lowfat	1 cup	130	16	1	10	3	1.5	15	125	0
whole milk	1 cup	149	11	1	9	8	5.0	32	113	0
Soy										
flavored, fruited	1 (6 oz.)	170	32	2	7	2	0.0	0	35	4
plain	1 cup	120	22	1 ½	5	3	0.0	0	30	1
Yoplait® Whips!®										
chocolate flavors	1 (4 oz.)	160	25	1 ½	5	3	2.0	10	75	0
fruit flavors	1 (4 oz.)	140	25	1 ½	5	3	2.0	10	75	0

MILK & YOGURT
Yogurt Drinks & Squeeze Yogurts

ITEM	AMOUNT	CALORIES	CARBOHYDRATE (g)	CARBOHYDRATE CHOICES	PROTEIN (g)	FAT (g)	SATURATED FAT (g)	CHOLESTEROL (mg)	SODIUM (mg)	FIBER (g)
Yogurt Drinks & Squeeze Yogurts										
Drinkable yogurt	1 (10 fl. oz.)	230	40	2 ½	10	3	2.0	15	150	2
Drinkable yogurt,										
w/ artificial sweetener	1 (7 fl. oz.)	60	10	½	5	0	0.0	0	85	0
GoGurt®	1 (2.25 fl. oz.)	70	13	1	2	1	0.0	0	30	0
Yoplait® frozen smoothie										
blueberry pomegranate	8 fl. oz.	110	19	1	5	2	1.0	5	80	2
strawberry banana	8 fl. oz.	110	19	1	5	2	1.0	5	80	2
triple berry	8 fl. oz.	110	19	1	5	2	1.0	5	80	2

NUTS, SEEDS & PEANUT BUTTER

ITEM	AMOUNT	CALORIES	CARBOHYDRATE (g)	CARBOHYDRATE CHOICES	PROTEIN (g)	FAT (g)	SATURATED FAT (g)	CHOLESTEROL (mg)	SODIUM (mg)	FIBER (g)
Almond butter	1 T.	99	3	0	2	9	1.0	0	70	1
Almond paste	1 T.	65	7	½	1	4	0.5	0	1	1
Almonds	23	160	6	½	6	14	1.0	0	0	3
Brazilnuts	8	230	4	0	5	23	5.5	0	1	3
Cashew butter	1 T.	94	4	0	3	8	1.5	0	98	0
Cashews, salted	23	170	8	½	5	13	2.0	0	115	1
Chestnuts	3	62	13	1	1	1	0.0	0	1	1
Filberts/hazelnuts	20	176	5	0	4	17	1.0	0	0	3
Flax seeds	2 T.	104	6	0	4	8	0.5	0	6	5
Hickory nuts	10	197	6	½	4	19	2.0	0	0	2
Macadamias	11	204	4	0	2	22	3.5	0	1	2
Mixed nuts										
w/ peanuts, salted	30	170	5	0	6	15	2.0	0	110	2
w/o peanuts, salted	20	170	6	½	5	15	2.5	0	105	2
Nutella® hazelnut spread	2 T.	200	22	1 ½	3	11	3.5	0	15	1
Peanut butter										
chunky	2 T.	190	7	½	7	16	3.0	0	120	2
creamy	2 T.	190	7	½	7	16	3.0	0	150	2
natural	2 T.	190	7	½	8	16	2.0	0	125	3
reduced fat	2 T.	200	12	1	9	12	2.0	0	120	2
Peanuts										
Beer Nuts®	39	170	7	½	7	14	3.0	0	80	2
dry roasted, salted	39	170	5	0	7	14	2.0	0	190	2
honey roasted	39	160	8	½	6	13	2.0	0	115	2
w/ oil, salted	39	170	6	½	7	14	2.0	0	115	2
Pecans	20 halves	196	4	0	3	20	2.0	0	0	3
Pine nuts	¼ cup	200	5	0	3	18	4.0	0	10	4
Pistachio nuts, salted	32	190	7	½	6	16	2.0	0	220	3
Poppy seeds	1 T.	45	2	0	2	4	0.5	0	2	1
Pumpkin/squash seeds	2 T.	36	4	0	2	2	0.5	0	46	0
Sesame butter/tahini	1 T.	89	3	0	3	8	1.0	0	5	1

NUTS, SEEDS, & PEANUT BUTTER

ITEM	AMOUNT	CALORIES	CARBOHYDRATE (g)	CARBOHYDRATE CHOICES	PROTEIN (g)	FAT (g)	SATURATED FAT (g)	CHOLESTEROL (mg)	SODIUM (mg)	FIBER (g)
Sesame seeds	2 T.	103	4	0	3	9	1.5	0	2	2
Soynut butter	2 T.	170	10	½	7	11	1.5	0	140	3
Soynuts, salted	3 T.	150	11	½	11	8	1.0	0	100	5
Sunflower seeds, salted	2 T.	100	4	0	3	9	1.0	0	69	2
Trail mix										
w/ chocolate chips	¼ cup	177	16	1	5	12	2.0	2	10	2
w/ fruit, tropical	¼ cup	143	23	1 ½	2	6	3.0	0	4	2
w/ seeds	¼ cup	173	17	1	5	11	2.0	0	86	2
Walnuts, chopped	2 T.	97	2	0	4	9	0.5	0	0	1

PASTA, RICE & OTHER GRAINS
(Cooked unless indicated.)
Pasta

ITEM	AMOUNT	CALORIES	CARBOHYDRATE (g)	CARBOHYDRATE CHOICES	PROTEIN (g)	FAT (g)	SATURATED FAT (g)	CHOLESTEROL (mg)	SODIUM (mg)	FIBER (g)
Cellophane noodles, dry	1 cup	200	50	3	0	0	0.0	0	0	0
Chow mein noodles, can	1 cup	260	38	2 ½	6	10	3.0	0	460	2
Couscous	1 cup	220	46	3	8	1	0.0	0	5	2
Egg noodles	1 cup	220	40	2 ½	8	3	1.0	70	15	2
Gnocchi, potato	1 cup	214	44	3	5	1	0.0	0	830	4
Macaroni/pasta										
regular	1 cup	210	42	3	7	1	0.0	0	0	2
whole wheat	1 cup	210	41	2 ½	7	2	0.0	0	4	5
Pastina	1 cup	210	42	3	7	1	0.0	0	0	2
Ramen noodles, w/ seasoning	1 cup	190	26	2	5	7	3.5	0	790	1
Ravioli, w/o sauce										
beef	9 (2 inch)	240	40	2 ½	9	4	1.5	10	280	2
cheese	9 (2 inch)	230	37	2 ½	10	4	2.0	15	290	2
Rice noodles	1 cup	192	44	3	2	0	0.0	0	33	2
Soba noodles	1 cup	113	24	1 ½	6	0	0.0	0	68	1
Spaghetti	1 cup	210	42	3	7	1	0.0	0	0	2
Tortellini, w/o sauce										
beef	28 small	320	40	2 ½	16	6	2.0	20	270	1
cheese	28 small	260	48	3	10	3	1.5	5	530	2

Rice

ITEM	AMOUNT	CALORIES	CARBOHYDRATE (g)	CARBOHYDRATE CHOICES	PROTEIN (g)	FAT (g)	SATURATED FAT (g)	CHOLESTEROL (mg)	SODIUM (mg)	FIBER (g)
Basmati	1 cup	170	37	2 ½	4	1	0.0	0	0	3
Brown										
instant	1 cup	170	36	2 ½	4	1	0.0	0	0	2
regular	1 cup	170	35	2	4	1	0.0	0	0	2
Pilaf	1 cup	220	43	3	2	4	2.0	10	810	1
Rice A Roni®, chicken										
reduced sodium	1 cup	270	51	3 ½	7	5	1.0	0	670	2
regular	1 cup	300	50	3	7	9	2.0	0	1060	3

PASTA, RICE & OTHER GRAINS

Rice

ITEM	AMOUNT	CALORIES	CARBOHYDRATE (g)	CARBOHYDRATE CHOICES	PROTEIN (g)	FAT (g)	SATURATED FAT (g)	CHOLESTEROL (mg)	SODIUM (mg)	FIBER (g)
Risotto	1 cup	150	37	2 ½	3	0	0.0	0	0	0
Spanish	1 cup	180	41	3	4	0	0.0	0	750	0
White										
instant	1 cup	190	43	3	3	1	0.0	0	15	0
regular	1 cup	170	38	2 ½	4	0	0.0	0	0	0
Wild	1 cup	170	35	2	6	0	0.0	0	0	2

Other Grains

ITEM	AMOUNT	CALORIES	CARBOHYDRATE (g)	CARBOHYDRATE CHOICES	PROTEIN (g)	FAT (g)	SATURATED FAT (g)	CHOLESTEROL (mg)	SODIUM (mg)	FIBER (g)
Barley										
pearled	½ cup	97	22	1 ½	2	0	0.0	0	2	3
whole	½ cup	135	30	2	4	1	0.0	0	1	7
Buckwheat/kasha	½ cup	77	17	1	3	1	0.0	0	3	2
Bulgur	½ cup	76	17	1	3	0	0.0	0	5	4
Millet	½ cup	104	21	1 ½	3	1	0.0	0	2	1
Polenta										
fried, slice, w/ oil	1 (4 oz.)	199	16	1	2	14	2.0	0	300	0
fried, slice, w/o oil	1 (4 oz.)	80	16	1	2	0	0.0	0	300	0
w/ water	1 cup	140	32	2	3	0	0.0	0	0	4
Quinoa, dry	¼ cup	160	29	2	6	3	0.5	0	9	3
Semolina, dry	1 T.	120	25	1 ½	3	0	0.0	0	0	0

POULTRY

Chicken

ITEM	AMOUNT	CALORIES	CARBOHYDRATE (g)	CARBOHYDRATE CHOICES	PROTEIN (g)	FAT (g)	SATURATED FAT (g)	CHOLESTEROL (mg)	SODIUM (mg)	FIBER (g)
Breasts										
BBQ, w/ skin	3 oz.	187	4	0	25	7	2.0	71	273	0
breaded & fried, w/ skin	3 oz.	221	8	½	21	11	3.0	72	234	0
deli	1 oz.	33	1	0	5	1	0.5	14	338	0
fried, w/ skin, w/ flour	3 oz.	189	1	0	27	8	2.0	76	65	0
fried, w/o skin	3 oz.	159	0	0	28	4	1.0	77	67	0
roasted, w/ skin	3 oz.	168	0	0	25	7	2.0	71	60	0
roasted, w/o skin	3 oz.	140	0	0	26	3	1.0	72	63	0
Capon, roasted, w/ skin	3 oz.	195	0	0	25	10	3.0	73	42	0
Cornish hens										
roasted, w/ skin	3 oz.	221	0	0	19	16	4.5	111	54	0
roasted, w/o skin	3 oz.	114	0	0	20	3	1.0	90	54	0
Giblets, fried	3 oz.	236	4	0	28	11	3.0	379	96	0
Gizzards, simmered	3 oz.	124	0	0	26	2	1.0	315	48	0
Hearts, simmered	3 oz.	157	0	0	23	7	2.0	206	41	0
Hot dogs	1 (1.6 oz.)	116	3	0	6	9	2.5	46	617	0
Legs										
breaded & fried, w/ skin	3 oz.	232	7	½	19	14	3.5	77	237	0
fried, w/ skin, w/ flour	3 oz.	216	2	0	23	12	3.5	80	75	0

POULTRY
Chicken

ITEM	AMOUNT	CALORIES	CARBOHYDRATE (g)	CARBOHYDRATE CHOICES	PROTEIN (g)	FAT (g)	SATURATED FAT (g)	CHOLESTEROL (mg)	SODIUM (mg)	FIBER (g)
Chicken legs *(continued)*										
fried, w/o skin	3 oz.	177	1	0	24	8	2.0	84	82	0
roasted, w/ skin	3 oz.	197	0	0	22	11	3.0	78	74	0
roasted, w/o skin	3 oz.	146	0	0	24	5	1.5	79	81	0
Livers, simmered	3 oz.	142	1	0	21	6	2.0	479	65	0
Pâté, chicken liver, can	1 oz.	57	2	0	4	4	1.0	111	109	0
Patties, breaded & fried	1 (3 oz.)	228	14	1	11	13	3.0	24	588	1
Strips, breaded & fried	4 (1.6 oz.)	504	37	2 ½	31	26	5.0	72	920	0
Thighs										
breaded & fried, w/ skin	3 oz.	248	9	½	17	15	4.0	95	434	1
fried, w/ skin, w/ flour	3 oz.	223	3	0	23	13	3.5	83	75	0
fried, w/o skin	3 oz.	185	1	0	24	9	2.5	87	81	0
roasted, w/ skin	3 oz.	210	0	0	21	13	3.5	79	71	0
roasted, w/o skin	3 oz.	166	0	0	21	8	2.5	77	64	0
Wings										
fried, w/ skin, w/ flour	1 (1 oz.)	91	1	0	7	6	1.5	23	22	0
roasted, w/ skin	1 (1 oz.)	82	0	0	8	6	1.5	24	23	0
Game										
Duck										
roasted, w/ skin	3 oz.	287	0	0	16	24	8.0	71	50	0
roasted, w/o skin	3 oz.	171	0	0	20	10	3.5	76	55	0
Goose										
roasted, w/ skin	3 oz.	259	0	0	21	19	6.0	77	60	0
roasted, w/o skin	3 oz.	202	0	0	25	11	4.0	82	65	0
Ostrich										
ground	3 oz.	149	0	0	22	6	1.5	71	68	0
tenderloin	3 oz.	140	0	0	25	4	1.0	91	98	0
Pheasant										
roasted, w/ skin	3 oz.	205	0	0	26	11	3.0	81	45	0
roasted, w/o skin	3 oz.	151	0	0	27	4	1.5	75	42	0
Quail										
roasted, w/ skin	3 oz.	218	0	0	22	14	4.0	86	60	0
roasted, w/o skin	3 oz.	152	0	0	25	5	1.5	79	58	0
Turkey										
Bacon	2 (1 oz.) slices	70	0	0	4	6	2.0	30	380	0
Bologna	1 oz.	59	1	0	3	5	1.0	21	355	0
Breast, deli	1 oz.	30	1	0	5	1	0.0	12	288	0
Dark meat										
roasted, w/ skin	3 oz.	184	0	0	24	9	3.0	77	68	0
roasted, w/o skin	3 oz.	157	0	0	24	6	2.0	75	70	0

POULTRY

Turkey

ITEM	AMOUNT	CALORIES	CARBOHYDRATE (g)	CARBOHYDRATE CHOICES	PROTEIN (g)	FAT (g)	SATURATED FAT (g)	CHOLESTEROL (mg)	SODIUM (mg)	FIBER (g)
Ground										
extra lean	3 oz.	120	0	0	28	2	0.5	45	65	0
lean	3 oz.	169	0	0	20	9	2.5	90	107	0
Ham, deli	1 oz.	32	0	0	5	1	0.5	19	320	0
Hot dogs	1 (1.6 oz.)	102	1	0	6	8	2.5	48	642	0
Light meat										
roasted, w/ skin	3 oz.	140	0	0	25	4	1.0	81	49	0
roasted, w/o skin	3 oz.	119	0	0	26	1	0.5	73	48	0
Pastrami, deli	1 oz.	35	1	0	5	1	0.5	19	278	0
Patties, breaded & fried	1 (3 oz.)	241	13	1	12	15	4.0	64	680	0
Sausages	1 (2 oz.)	93	0	0	11	6	1.5	43	470	0

RESTAURANT FAVORITES

Appetizers

ITEM	AMOUNT	CALORIES	CARBOHYDRATE (g)	CARBOHYDRATE CHOICES	PROTEIN (g)	FAT (g)	SATURATED FAT (g)	CHOLESTEROL (mg)	SODIUM (mg)	FIBER (g)
Breadsticks	1 medium	140	26	2	5	2	0.0	0	270	1
Bruschetta	1 (4 inch)	62	6	½	2	4	1.0	2	125	0
Buffalo wings	4	210	4	0	22	12	3.0	130	900	0
Clams casino	6	377	19	1	35	17	10.0	115	802	1
Crab cakes, fried	1 (4 oz.)	290	20	1	9	19	4.0	149	893	0
Cream cheese puffs	3	331	14	1	3	29	6.5	18	180	0
Focaccia bread	1 (6 inch)	271	47	3	7	6	1.0	0	446	3
Garlic bread	1 (4 inch)	322	38	2 ½	12	14	4.0	20	522	4
Jalapeño poppers	6	360	32	2	7	22	10.0	45	810	3
Mozzarella sticks, w/ sauce	4	378	28	2	19	22	12.0	24	2712	3
Mushrooms, fried	8	237	13	1	4	19	3.0	22	193	1
Nachos, deluxe	1 order	1048	91	5 ½	46	57	23.0	109	2252	17
Oysters Rockefeller	6	170	10	½	8	10	2.0	46	392	0
Pork dumplings, fried	1 (3.5 oz.)	340	24	1 ½	13	21	6.0	29	346	1
Potato skins	6	500	30	2	20	34	14.0	80	1020	8
Shrimp cocktail, w/ sauce	5	42	3	0	6	0	0.0	54	262	1
Spring rolls, w/ meat	1 (2.5 oz.)	127	10	½	6	7	2.0	41	336	1
Stuffed mushrooms	3	134	10	½	4	9	5.0	23	183	1
Wontons, w/ meat	1 (0.7 oz.)	61	4	0	3	4	0.5	13	83	0

Desserts

ITEM	AMOUNT	CALORIES	CARBOHYDRATE (g)	CARBOHYDRATE CHOICES	PROTEIN (g)	FAT (g)	SATURATED FAT (g)	CHOLESTEROL (mg)	SODIUM (mg)	FIBER (g)
Apple pie à la mode	1 (6 oz.)	433	58	4	5	21	8.0	29	292	2
Caramel apple bars	1 (5 oz.)	370	54	3 ½	4	18	3.0	25	200	1
Carrot cake, w/ icing	1 (4 oz.)	494	53	3 ½	5	30	6.0	61	279	1
Cheesecake	1 (3 oz.)	295	23	1 ½	5	21	11.0	51	190	0
Chocolate chip cookies	1 (2 oz.)	280	40	2 ½	3	13	8.0	40	85	2
Chocolate mousse cake	1 (3 oz.)	291	41	3	2	12	4.0	29	140	2
Chocolate peanut butter pie	1 (6 oz.)	653	64	4	12	39	19.0	27	319	3

RESTAURANT FAVORITES

Desserts

ITEM	AMOUNT	CALORIES	CARBOHYDRATE (g)	CARBOHYDRATE CHOICES	PROTEIN (g)	FAT (g)	SATURATED FAT (g)	CHOLESTEROL (mg)	SODIUM (mg)	FIBER (g)
Crème brûlée	¾ cup	347	35	2	7	20	11.0	311	125	0
Fortune cookies	1	30	7	½	0	0	0.0	0	22	0
Fudge brownie sundae	1 (8 oz.)	687	83	5 ½	9	38	11.0	62	486	3
Key lime pie	1 (4.5 oz.)	410	59	4	5	17	11.0	15	290	1
Smoothie	1 (16 fl. oz.)	320	70	4 ½	7	1	0.5	5	160	4
Tiramisu	1 (5 oz.)	368	33	2	9	22	13.0	187	291	0

Entrées
American

ITEM	AMOUNT	CALORIES	CARBOHYDRATE (g)	CARBOHYDRATE CHOICES	PROTEIN (g)	FAT (g)	SATURATED FAT (g)	CHOLESTEROL (mg)	SODIUM (mg)	FIBER (g)
Baked potato, w/ broccoli & cheese	1 (10 oz.)	1168	114	7	28	71	18.0	52	1684	16
BBQ beef sandwich	1 (6.5 oz.)	392	39	2 ½	20	17	6.0	54	1056	3
BBQ pork sandwich	1 (6.5 oz.)	347	39	2 ½	23	10	3.0	52	889	3
BBQ ribs	8 oz.	700	36	2 ½	44	42	18.0	130	1240	0
Chicken fried steak	8 oz.	530	28	2	30	34	16.0	54	1336	2
Filet mignon	8 oz.	479	0	0	64	23	8.5	191	143	0
Fried shrimp	12 large	218	10	½	19	11	2.0	159	310	0
Grilled salmon	8 oz.	423	0	0	59	19	3.0	135	2365	0
King crab legs	9 oz.	248	0	0	50	4	0.0	135	2735	0
Prime rib	12 oz.	1334	0	0	74	113	47.0	289	211	0
Shrimp Creole, w/ rice	2 cups	611	51	3 ½	55	19	4.0	371	1310	3
Shrimp jambalaya	2 cups	611	51	3 ½	55	19	4.0	371	1310	3
Southwestern tuna wrap	1 (14 oz.)	950	53	3 ½	41	64	17.0	110	1230	4
Stuffed shrimp	2 cups	552	17	1	56	27	6.0	443	1388	1
T-bone steak	10 oz.	530	0	0	42	40	18.0	121	534	0
Turkey & cheese bagel	1 (11 oz.)	506	66	4 ½	34	11	5.5	56	1393	4

Asian/Chinese

ITEM	AMOUNT	CALORIES	CARBOHYDRATE (g)	CARBOHYDRATE CHOICES	PROTEIN (g)	FAT (g)	SATURATED FAT (g)	CHOLESTEROL (mg)	SODIUM (mg)	FIBER (g)
Beef & broccoli	2 cups	512	14	1	76	39	10.0	202	1473	5
Cashew chicken	2 cups	817	29	1 ½	54	57	9.5	121	1975	4
Chicken curry	2 cups	586	20	1	54	32	7.0	168	2376	4
Egg rolls, meatless	1 (2.5 oz.)	113	11	1	3	6	1.5	33	339	1
Kung Pao chicken	2 cups	818	22	1 ½	54	58	10.0	120	1976	4
Pork chow mein, w/ noodles	2 cups	869	62	4	44	51	10.5	96	1631	7
Shrimp & snow peas	2 cups	439	19	1	38	23	3.0	295	2134	3
Stir-fry chicken & fried rice	2 cups	432	45	3	19	19	3.5	85	853	3
Sushi, w/ fish & vegetables	1 cup	238	48	3	9	1	0.0	11	344	1
Sushi rolls										
fish, w/ rice	1 small	47	8	½	2	1	0.5	7	38	0
vegetarian, w/ rice	1 small	31	6	½	1	0	0.0	0	23	0
Sweet & sour pork, w/ rice	2 cups	537	79	5	26	13	3.5	57	1813	3
Tofu & vegetable stir-fry	2 cups	293	34	2	15	14	2.0	0	445	10

RESTAURANT FAVORITES

Entrées - Italian/Mediterranean

ITEM	AMOUNT	CALORIES	CARBOHYDRATE (g)	CARBOHYDRATE CHOICES	PROTEIN (g)	FAT (g)	SATURATED FAT (g)	CHOLESTEROL (mg)	SODIUM (mg)	FIBER (g)
Italian/Mediterranean										
Calzones, w/ pepperoni	1 (6 oz.)	450	49	3	21	19	9.0	10	930	6
Chicken cacciatore	2 cups	916	26	2	84	51	13.0	320	1183	4
Chicken cordon bleu	8 oz.	483	9	½	46	28	15.0	191	489	1
Chicken Marsala	8 oz.	593	12	1	55	31	11.0	177	540	1
Chicken/veal parmigiana	8 oz.	466	29	2	36	23	8.0	115	929	1
Eggs Benedict	19 oz.	860	55	3 ½	35	56	23.0	525	1943	3
Fettuccini Alfredo	2 cups	1430	68	4 ½	31	119	71.0	340	1470	3
Gyros	½ pita	296	23	1 ½	15	15	7.5	55	604	1
Linguini, w/ pesto sauce	2 cups	706	83	5	23	31	7.0	18	425	6
Lobster Newburg	2 cups	1225	23	1 ½	60	100	59.0	738	1294	0
Moussaka	2 cups	474	26	1 ½	33	26	9.0	193	863	7
Pasta, w/ carbonara sauce	2 cups	651	83	5	25	24	10.5	93	496	5
Pasta, w/ marinara sauce	2 cups	530	94	6	17	9	1.0	0	1100	10
Seafood Alfredo	2 cups	1014	62	4	38	69	41.0	337	672	5
Shrimp scampi	2 cups	438	2	0	58	20	10.0	480	584	0
Spanakopita	8 oz.	387	37	2 ½	16	20	10.0	227	769	4
Stuffed grape leaves	4	212	7	½	7	17	4.0	52	65	1
Veal scallopini	8 oz.	608	2	0	42	46	13.0	146	900	0
Vegetarian lasagna	2 cups	720	70	4 ½	40	34	24.0	130	1740	4
Mexican										
Chimichangas, beef & cheese	1 (6.5 oz.)	443	39	2 ½	20	23	11.0	51	957	0
Enchiladas										
cheese	2 (6 inch)	639	57	4	19	38	21.0	88	1568	1
seafood	2 (6 inch)	529	43	3	25	29	17.0	83	1372	1
Fajitas										
chicken	1 (9 oz.)	520	53	3 ½	18	26	8.0	70	1300	4
steak	1 (9 oz.)	510	52	3 ½	21	25	8.0	50	1200	3
Huevos rancheros	1 (2 egg)	410	24	1 ½	23	26	9.5	450	530	4
Quesadillas	1 (2 oz.)	199	21	1 ½	6	10	3.5	14	255	1
Rice & beans	2 cups	520	84	5	20	12	4.0	20	1440	12
Salads, w/ dressing										
Caesar	4 cups	338	20	1	8	25	5.0	7	725	3
Chicken Caesar	4 cups	655	23	1 ½	37	47	9.0	86	1728	4
Greek	1 (14 oz.)	441	18	1	13	37	14.0	67	1301	4
Niçoise	1 (12 oz.)	423	26	1 ½	19	28	4.0	36	1026	5
Oriental chicken	1 (9 oz.)	270	17	1	40	4	0.5	70	700	5
Tossed, w/ gorgonzola	4 cups	400	9	½	20	34	13.0	50	800	3

RESTAURANT FAVORITES
Side Dishes

ITEM	AMOUNT	CALORIES	CARBOHYDRATE (g)	CARBOHYDRATE CHOICES	PROTEIN (g)	FAT (g)	SATURATED FAT (g)	CHOLESTEROL (mg)	SODIUM (mg)	FIBER (g)
Side Dishes										
Garlic mashed potatoes	1 cup	209	18	1	3	14	8.0	33	132	3
Grilled vegetables	1½ cups	120	15	1	6	4	0.0	0	310	3
Oven roasted potatoes	1½ cups	260	50	3	6	6	1.0	0	300	4
Polenta	½ cup	163	21	1 ½	4	8	3.0	12	571	2
Ratatouille	1 cup	133	12	1	1	10	1.5	0	106	4
Risotto	½ cup	281	29	2	7	15	9.0	36	851	1
Soft pretzels	1 large	340	72	5	10	1	0.0	0	900	3
Soups										
Borscht	1 cup	73	7	½	3	4	2.5	8	498	2
Cheese	1 cup	626	28	2	36	42	26.0	132	1464	2
Chicken chili	1 cup	233	21	1 ½	14	12	7.0	43	1353	4
Chilled fruit	1 cup	99	25	1 ½	1	0	0.0	0	12	1
Clam chowder	1 cup	270	16	1	11	20	9.0	63	730	1
Egg drop	1 cup	73	1	0	8	4	1.0	103	729	0
French onion, w/ croutons	1 cup	260	27	2	12	12	6.0	18	1020	2
Gazpacho	1 cup	68	10	½	2	3	0.0	0	286	2
Hot & sour	1 cup	133	5	0	12	6	2.0	23	1563	0
Minestrone	1 cup	154	23	1 ½	6	5	0.5	0	790	4
Seafood stew	1 cup	173	9	½	23	5	1.0	95	359	2
Shrimp gumbo	1 cup	151	18	1	10	5	1.0	50	590	4
Tomato Florentine	1 cup	61	14	1	4	1	0.5	3	1035	3
Vichyssoise	1 cup	223	18	1	5	15	8.0	44	336	2
Wonton	1 cup	45	5	0	4	1	0.0	15	940	1

SALAD DRESSINGS

ITEM	AMOUNT	CALORIES	CARBOHYDRATE (g)	CARBOHYDRATE CHOICES	PROTEIN (g)	FAT (g)	SATURATED FAT (g)	CHOLESTEROL (mg)	SODIUM (mg)	FIBER (g)
Bleu cheese										
fat free	1 T.	18	4	0	0	0	0.0	0	140	0
light	1 T.	25	3	0	0	1	0.5	0	155	0
regular	1 T.	70	1	0	0	8	1.5	0	150	0
Buttermilk	1 T.	75	1	0	0	8	1.0	3	120	0
Caesar										
fat free	1 T.	25	6	½	0	0	0.0	0	175	0
light	1 T.	35	2	0	1	3	0.5	0	310	0
regular	1 T.	85	1	0	0	10	1.5	3	80	0
Caesar Italian, fat free	1 T.	13	5	0	0	0	0.0	0	235	0
Catalina										
fat free	1 T.	25	6	½	0	0	0.0	0	175	0
regular	1 T.	50	5	0	0	3	0.5	0	210	0
Chipotle ranch	1 T.	85	2	0	0	9	1.5	3	115	0
Creamy parmesan	1 T.	90	1	0	1	9	1.5	5	150	0

SALAD DRESSINGS

ITEM	AMOUNT	CALORIES	CARBOHYDRATE (g)	CARBOHYDRATE CHOICES	PROTEIN (g)	FAT (g)	SATURATED FAT (g)	CHOLESTEROL (mg)	SODIUM (mg)	FIBER (g)
French										
fat free	1 T.	23	6	½	0	0	0.0	0	145	0
light	1 T.	25	4	0	0	1	0.0	0	125	0
regular	1 T.	65	3	0	0	6	1.0	0	135	0
Green Goddess®	1 T.	65	1	0	0	7	1.0	0	130	0
Honey mustard	1 T.	65	4	0	0	6	1.0	8	105	0
Italian										
creamy, regular	1 T.	55	2	0	0	5	1.0	0	120	0
fat free	1 T.	10	2	0	0	0	0.0	0	195	0
light	1 T.	18	2	0	0	1	0.0	0	155	0
regular	1 T.	35	2	0	0	3	0.5	0	155	0
regular, mix	1 T.	63	1	0	0	7	1.0	0	161	0
Oil & vinegar	1 T.	70	0	0	0	8	1.5	0	0	0
Peppercorn parmesan	1 T.	75	2	0	1	8	1.5	3	180	0
Peppercorn ranch, fat free	1 T.	25	6	½	0	0	0.0	0	175	0
Ranch										
fat free	1 T.	15	3	0	0	0	0.0	0	155	0
light	1 T.	40	2	0	1	4	0.5	3	145	0
regular	1 T.	70	1	0	1	7	1.5	5	130	0
Russian										
light	1 T.	23	5	0	0	1	0.0	1	142	0
regular	1 T.	60	7	½	0	3	0.5	0	180	0
Salad Spritzers®										
Balsamic Breeze	10 sprays	10	1	0	0	1	0.0	0	130	0
Caesar Delight®	10 sprays	10	1	0	0	1	0.0	0	85	0
Italian vinaigrette	10 sprays	10	1	0	0	1	0.0	0	100	0
Sesame seed	1 T.	68	1	0	1	7	1.0	0	153	0
Thousand island										
fat free	1 T.	20	5	0	0	0	0.0	0	140	1
light	1 T.	25	5	0	0	1	0.0	3	145	0
regular	1 T.	65	3	0	0	6	1.0	5	165	0
Vinaigrette										
balsamic, regular	1 T.	50	3	0	0	5	1.0	0	115	0
raspberry, light	1 T.	40	6	½	0	2	0.5	0	10	0
red wine, fat free	1 T.	15	4	0	0	0	0.0	0	115	0
red wine, light	1 T.	23	2	0	0	2	0.5	0	160	0
red wine, regular	1 T.	45	1	0	0	5	0.5	0	240	0
Western®										
fat free	1 T.	25	6	½	0	0	0.0	0	140	0
regular	1 T.	80	6	½	0	6	1.0	0	115	0

For mayonnaise/Miracle Whip®, see Fats, Oils, Cream & Gravy.

SALADS

ITEM	AMOUNT	CALORIES	CARBOHYDRATE (g)	CARBOHYDRATE CHOICES	PROTEIN (g)	FAT (g)	SATURATED FAT (g)	CHOLESTEROL (mg)	SODIUM (mg)	FIBER (g)
SALADS										
Caesar, w/ dressing	1 cup	204	7	½	7	17	4.5	14	453	1
Carrot-raisin	½ cup	202	21	1 ½	1	14	2.0	10	118	2
Chef										
w/ dressing	1 cup	312	9	½	17	23	7.5	111	924	2
w/o dressing	1 cup	178	3	0	17	11	5.5	93	496	2
Chicken, w/ mayo.	½ cup	268	1	0	11	25	3.0	48	201	0
Coleslaw										
w/ mayo.	½ cup	98	9	½	1	7	1.0	3	178	1
w/ vinaigrette	½ cup	41	7	½	1	2	0.0	5	14	1
Cucumber										
creamy, w/ mayo.	½ cup	59	5	0	1	4	3.0	9	13	1
w/ vinegar	½ cup	24	6	½	0	0	0.0	0	1	1
Egg, w/ mayo.	½ cup	292	1	0	8	28	5.5	290	232	0
Fruit, fresh	½ cup	51	13	1	1	0	0.0	0	0	2
Gelatin, w/ fruit	½ cup	73	18	1	1	0	0.0	0	30	1
Ham, w/ mayo.	½ cup	259	13	1	10	19	6.0	44	1094	0
Lobster, w/ mayo.	½ cup	75	5	0	6	4	0.5	56	157	1
Macaroni, w/ mayo.	½ cup	230	14	1	2	19	2.0	14	180	1
Pasta primavera	½ cup	152	26	2	4	4	1.0	0	311	2
Potato										
German-style	½ cup	136	20	1	2	5	2.0	8	470	1
w/ eggs & mayo.	½ cup	179	14	1	3	10	2.0	85	661	2
w/ mayo.	½ cup	138	17	1	2	8	1.0	6	105	2
Seafood										
w/ mayo.	½ cup	164	2	0	13	11	1.5	66	176	0
w/ pasta, vinaigrette	½ cup	126	11	1	5	7	1.0	17	524	1
Shrimp, w/ mayo.	½ cup	141	3	0	13	8	1.5	103	196	0
Spinach, w/o dressing	1 cup	108	11	1	5	5	1.5	77	227	2
Tabbouleh	2 T.	30	3	0	1	1	0.0	0	63	1
Taco										
w/ salsa	1 (16 oz.)	420	33	2	24	21	11.0	65	1400	11
w/ salsa & shell	1 (19 oz.)	790	73	4 ½	31	42	15.0	65	1670	13
Three bean, w/ oil	½ cup	70	7	½	2	4	0.5	0	260	3
Tortellini, cheese	½ cup	189	14	1	5	14	3.0	23	561	2
Tossed, w/o dressing	1 cup	26	5	0	2	0	0.0	0	25	2
Tuna, w/ mayo.	½ cup	192	10	½	16	9	1.5	13	412	0
Waldorf, w/ mayo.	½ cup	205	6	½	2	20	2.0	10	117	2

SOUPS
Canned, prepared

ITEM	AMOUNT	CALORIES	CARBOHYDRATE (g)	CARBOHYDRATE CHOICES	PROTEIN (g)	FAT (g)	SATURATED FAT (g)	CHOLESTEROL (mg)	SODIUM (mg)	FIBER (g)
SOUPS										
Canned, prepared										
Bean										
w/ bacon	1 cup	170	25	1 ½	8	4	1.5	5	860	8
w/ franks	1 cup	188	22	1	10	7	2.0	13	1093	6
Beef barley, w/ veg.	1 cup	90	15	1	5	2	1.0	10	890	3
Beef broth										
reduced sodium	1 cup	15	0	0	3	0	0.0	0	450	0
regular	1 cup	15	1	0	3	0	0.0	0	860	0
Beef consommé	1 cup	20	1	0	4	0	0.0	0	810	0
Beef noodle	1 cup	90	12	1	8	1	0.0	20	980	0
Black bean	1 cup	170	30	1 ½	8	2	0.0	3	730	10
Cheddar cheese*	1 cup	165	18	1	6	7	3.0	13	953	1
Chicken alphabet	1 cup	70	11	1	4	2	0.5	10	660	1
Chicken & dumplings	1 cup	96	6	½	6	6	1.5	34	860	1
Chicken & rice	1 cup	70	13	1	2	2	0.5	5	820	0
Chicken & stars	1 cup	70	10	½	3	2	0.5	5	640	1
Chicken broth										
reduced sodium	1 cup	15	0	0	3	0	0.0	0	570	0
regular	1 cup	15	0	0	1	1	0.0	0	930	0
Chicken gumbo	1 cup	60	10	½	2	1	0.5	5	870	1
Chicken noodle	1 cup	60	8	½	3	2	0.5	10	890	0
Chili beef, w/ beans	1 cup	170	21	1	7	7	3.5	13	1035	10
Chunky, Campbell's®										
chicken & dumplings	1 cup	160	16	1	7	8	2.0	30	890	3
chicken corn chowder	1 cup	140	22	1 ½	7	3	1.0	10	410	2
chicken noodle	1 cup	110	16	1	7	3	1.0	20	410	2
grilled chicken & sausage gumbo	1 cup	140	21	1 ½	8	3	1.0	15	410	3
hearty beef barley	1 cup	160	26	2	9	2	0.5	10	790	4
hearty Italian-style wedding	1 cup	160	24	1 ½	8	3	1.0	15	650	3
New England clam chowder	1 cup	130	20	1	5	3	1.0	10	410	2
savory chicken, w/ rice	1 cup	110	18	1	6	2	0.5	10	810	2
savory vegetable	1 cup	120	24	1 ½	3	1	0.5	0	410	4
sirloin burger, w/ veg.	1 cup	130	18	1	8	3	1.0	15	800	3
steak & potato	1 cup	120	18	1	7	2	0.5	15	890	3
Clam chowder										
Manhattan	1 cup	70	12	1	2	1	0.5	0	880	2
New England*	1 cup	145	19	1	8	5	1.5	13	956	1
Corn chowder*	1 cup	150	28	2	4	3	1.5	10	690	2
Cream of asparagus*	1 cup	165	15	1	6	9	2.5	13	893	3
Cream of broccoli*	1 cup	145	18	1	6	6	2.0	13	813	1
Cream of celery	1 cup	100	7	½	1	7	2.0	5	860	0

SOUPS
Canned, prepared

ITEM	AMOUNT	CALORIES	CARBOHYDRATE (g)	CARBOHYDRATE CHOICES	PROTEIN (g)	FAT (g)	SATURATED FAT (g)	CHOLESTEROL (mg)	SODIUM (mg)	FIBER (g)
Cream of chicken	1 cup	120	10	½	3	8	2.5	10	870	2
Cream of mushroom										
condensed, lowfat	½ cup	70	9	½	2	3	0.5	0	630	1
condensed, regular	½ cup	100	9	½	1	6	1.5	5	870	2
lowfat	1 cup	70	9	½	2	3	0.5	0	840	1
reduced sodium	1 cup	70	10	½	2	2	0.5	5	470	1
regular	1 cup	100	9	½	1	6	1.5	5	870	1
Cream of potato*	1 cup	145	21	1 ½	6	4	2.0	13	863	2
Cream of shrimp*	1 cup	145	14	1	6	7	2.0	18	941	1
Double Noodle®	1 cup	110	20	1	3	2	0.5	10	480	1
Escarole	1 cup	25	3	0	1	1	0.0	0	930	1
French onion	1 cup	45	6	½	2	2	1.0	0	900	1
Gazpacho	1 cup	46	4	0	7	0	0.0	0	739	0
Green pea	1 cup	180	28	2	9	3	1.0	0	870	4
Healthy Choice®										
cheese tortellini	1 cup	90	18	1	3	1	0.0	5	390	3
chicken noodle	1 cup	90	12	1	8	1	0.0	15	390	1
chicken w/ rice	1 cup	90	13	1	6	2	0.5	10	390	1
garden vegetable	1 cup	130	25	1 ½	5	1	1.0	5	450	5
red beans & rice	1 cup	150	27	1 ½	4	2	0.0	5	390	5
split pea & ham	1 cup	160	27	1 ½	12	3	1.0	10	470	6
tomato basil	1 cup	100	22	1 ½	2	0	0.0	0	450	3
vegetable beef	1 cup	130	21	1 ½	9	2	0.0	10	420	4
Healthy Request®										
chicken w/ whole grain pasta	1 cup	100	14	1	7	2	0.5	20	410	1
cream of mushroom	1 cup	70	10	½	2	2	0.5	5	410	1
homestyle chicken noodle	1 cup	60	10	½	3	2	0.5	10	410	1
Mexican-style chicken tortilla	1 cup	120	19	1	7	2	1.0	15	410	2
savory chicken & brown rice	1 cup	120	19	1	7	2	0.5	15	410	1
tomato	1 cup	90	17	1	2	2	0.5	0	410	1
vegetable beef	1 cup	90	15	1	5	1	0.0	5	410	3
Hot & sour	1 cup	162	5	0	15	8	2.5	34	1011	1
Italian-style wedding	1 cup	90	12	1	4	3	1.0	10	810	3
Lentil	1 cup	140	24	1 ½	9	1	0.5	0	800	6
Lobster bisque	1 cup	130	11	1	6	6	3.0	70	990	0
Matzo ball	1 cup	110	13	1	3	5	2.0	35	710	3
Minestrone	1 cup	90	17	1	4	1	0.5	0	960	3
Mushroom	1 cup	80	10	½	2	4	1.0	5	890	1
Oyster stew*	1 cup	135	11	1	6	8	4.5	28	973	0
Pasta e fagioli	1 cup	170	19	1	7	7	2.5	10	1040	4
Pepper pot	1 cup	90	9	½	4	4	1.5	20	940	1
Scotch broth	1 cup	70	9	½	3	2	1.0	5	880	2

SOUPS
Canned, prepared

ITEM	AMOUNT	CALORIES	CARBOHYDRATE (g)	CARBOHYDRATE CHOICES	PROTEIN (g)	FAT (g)	SATURATED FAT (g)	CHOLESTEROL (mg)	SODIUM (mg)	FIBER (g)
Seafood chowder*	1 cup	131	15	1	11	3	1.0	20	692	0
Split pea, w/ ham	1 cup	180	27	1 ½	10	4	2.0	5	850	5
Tomato										
bisque*	1 cup	179	27	2	6	6	3.0	20	1002	1
creamy, ready to serve	1 cup	100	17	1	2	2	1.5	10	690	4
reduced sodium	1 cup	90	20	1	2	0	0.0	0	530	1
regular, w/ milk*	1 cup	145	26	2	6	2	1.0	8	773	1
regular, w/ water	1 cup	90	20	1	2	0	0.0	0	710	1
w/ rice, w/ water	1 cup	119	22	1 ½	2	3	0.5	3	815	2
Turkey noodle	1 cup	64	8	½	4	2	0.5	5	758	1
Vegetable	1 cup	82	13	1	3	2	0.5	2	810	0
Vegetable beef	1 cup	80	15	1	5	1	0.5	5	890	3
Vegetable broth	1 cup	25	6	½	0	0	0.0	0	590	0
Vegetarian vegetable	1 cup	90	18	1	3	1	0.0	0	790	2
Wild rice, w/ chicken	1 cup	70	12	1	3	2	0.5	5	820	1

*Prepared w/ ½ cup 1% milk. If prepared w/ whole milk add 20 calories, 3 g fat, and 12 mg cholesterol. If prepared w/ skim milk subtract 15 calories and 2 g fat.

Dehydrated/Boxed *(Prepared unless indicated.)*

ITEM	AMOUNT	CALORIES	CARBOHYDRATE (g)	CARBOHYDRATE CHOICES	PROTEIN (g)	FAT (g)	SATURATED FAT (g)	CHOLESTEROL (mg)	SODIUM (mg)	FIBER (g)
Beef noodle	1 cup	40	6	½	2	1	0.0	3	1035	1
Bouillon, regular, dry										
beef	1 cube	5	0	0	0	0	0.0	0	900	0
chicken	1 cube	5	0	0	0	0	0.0	0	1100	0
vegetable	1 cube	5	0	0	0	0	0.0	0	960	0
Bouillon, sodium-free, dry										
beef	1 tsp.	10	2	0	0	0	0.0	0	0	0
chicken	1 tsp.	10	2	0	0	0	0.0	0	0	0
Chicken noodle	1 cup	70	12	1	3	2	0.0	15	690	0
Chicken rice	1 cup	58	9	½	2	1	0.5	2	931	1
Cream of vegetable	1 cup	107	12	1	2	6	1.5	0	1171	1
Cup-a-Soup®										
chicken noodle	1 (6 oz.)	50	8	½	2	1	0.0	10	540	0
cream of chicken	1 (6 oz.)	60	12	1	0	2	0.0	0	640	0
tomato	1 (6 oz.)	90	19	1	2	1	0.0	0	520	0
Cup Noodles®										
beef	1 (14 oz.)	300	38	2 ½	7	13	7.0	0	1110	2
chicken	1 (14 oz.)	300	38	2 ½	6	13	7.0	0	1060	2
Leek	1 cup	60	11	1	2	1	0.0	0	770	0
Minestrone	1 cup	100	20	1	4	1	0.0	0	590	2
Miso	1 cup	35	4	0	2	1	0.0	0	800	1
Mushroom	1 cup	96	11	1	2	5	1.0	0	1020	1
Onion	1 cup	35	6	½	1	1	0.0	0	920	0

SOUPS
Dehydrated/Boxed

ITEM	AMOUNT	CALORIES	CARBOHYDRATE (g)	CARBOHYDRATE CHOICES	PROTEIN (g)	FAT (g)	SATURATED FAT (g)	CHOLESTEROL (mg)	SODIUM (mg)	FIBER (g)
Onion soup mix, dry	1 T.	20	4	0	0	0	0.0	0	610	0
Ramen noodle										
beef	1 cup	190	26	2	5	7	3.5	0	790	1
chicken	1 cup	190	26	2	5	7	3.5	0	790	1
shrimp	1 cup	190	26	2	5	7	3.5	0	860	1
Tomato	1 cup	103	19	1	3	2	1.0	0	943	1
Vegetable	1 cup	25	6	½	1	0	0.0	0	530	0
Vegetable beef	1 cup	53	8	½	3	1	0.5	0	1002	1

VEGETABLES
(For dried beans, peas and lentils, see Vegetarian Foods & Legumes.)

ITEM	AMOUNT	CALORIES	CARBOHYDRATE (g)	CARBOHYDRATE CHOICES	PROTEIN (g)	FAT (g)	SATURATED FAT (g)	CHOLESTEROL (mg)	SODIUM (mg)	FIBER (g)
Alfalfa sprouts, raw	½ cup	4	0	0	1	0	0.0	0	1	0
Artichokes										
boiled/steamed	1 medium	60	14	½	4	0	0.0	0	120	7
hearts, marinated	½ cup	58	7	½	2	4	0.0	0	24	42
Asparagus, cooked	½ cup	20	4	0	2	0	0.0	0	13	2
Bamboo shoots, raw	½ cup	20	4	0	2	0	0.0	0	3	2
Bean sprouts, raw	½ cup	0	16	3	2	0	0.0	0	3	1
Beets, pickled	½ cup	74	19	1	1	0	0.0	0	300	3
Bok choy, cooked	½ cup	10	2	0	1	0	0.0	0	29	1
Broccoli										
cooked	½ cup	26	5	0	3	0	0.0	0	10	3
florets, raw	½ cup	10	2	0	1	0	0.0	0	10	1
w/ cheese sauce, cooked	½ cup	90	8	½	3	5	3.0	5	490	1
Brussel sprouts, cooked	½ cup	28	6	½	2	0	0.0	0	16	2
Cabbage										
Chinese, cooked	½ cup	11	2	0	1	0	0.0	0	55	1
green, cooked	½ cup	17	4	0	1	0	0.0	0	6	1
red, raw	½ cup	11	3	0	1	0	0.0	0	10	1
Carrots										
cooked	½ cup	27	6	½	1	0	0.0	0	45	2
raw	1 large	30	7	½	1	0	0.0	0	50	2
Cauliflower										
cooked	½ cup	14	3	0	1	0	0.0	0	9	1
raw	½ cup	13	3	0	1	0	0.0	0	15	1
w/ cheese sauce, cooked	½ cup	45	5	0	2	2	0.5	5	310	1
Celery										
cooked	½ cup	12	3	0	1	0	0.0	0	65	1
raw	1 medium	6	1	0	0	0	0.0	0	32	1
Chinese-style, frzn.	½ cup	40	8	½	1	1	0.0	0	10	2
Chives, raw	1 T.	1	0	0	0	0	0.0	0	0	0

VEGETABLES

ITEM	AMOUNT	CALORIES	CARBOHYDRATE (g)	CARBOHYDRATE CHOICES	PROTEIN (g)	FAT (g)	SATURATED FAT (g)	CHOLESTEROL (mg)	SODIUM (mg)	FIBER (g)
Corn, cooked										
cream-style, can	½ cup	92	23	1 ½	2	1	0.0	0	365	2
on the cob	1 (4 oz.)	123	29	2	4	2	0.0	0	19	3
w/ butter sauce, frzn.	½ cup	150	28	2	3	3	1.0	0	260	2
whole kernel, can	½ cup	66	15	1	2	1	0.0	0	244	2
whole kernel, frzn.	½ cup	66	16	1	2	1	0.0	0	1	2
Cucumbers, raw										
w/ skin	½ large	23	6	½	1	0	0.0	0	3	1
w/o skin	½ large	17	3	0	1	0	0.0	0	3	1
Eggplant, cooked	½ cup	17	4	0	0	0	0.0	0	1	1
Endive, raw	1 cup	9	2	0	1	0	0.0	0	11	2
Green beans, cooked										
French-style	½ cup	15	3	0	1	0	0.0	0	0	1
snap	½ cup	22	5	0	1	0	0.0	0	1	2
Green onions, raw	¼ cup	8	2	0	1	0	0.0	0	4	1
Greens, cooked										
beet	½ cup	19	4	0	2	0	0.0	0	174	2
collard	½ cup	21	4	0	2	0	0.0	0	13	2
dandelion	½ cup	17	3	0	1	0	0.0	0	23	2
mustard	½ cup	11	2	0	2	0	0.0	0	11	1
turnip	½ cup	14	3	0	1	0	0.0	0	21	3
Hominy, cooked	½ cup	58	11	1	1	1	0.0	0	168	2
Italian-style, frzn.	½ cup	20	3	0	1	0	0.0	0	23	1
Jicama, cooked/raw	½ cup	25	6	½	1	0	0.0	0	3	3
Kale, cooked	½ cup	18	4	0	1	0	0.0	0	15	1
Kohlrabi, cooked	½ cup	24	6	½	2	0	0.0	0	17	1
Leeks, raw	¼ cup	14	3	0	0	0	0.0	0	4	0
Lettuce, raw	1 cup	8	2	0	1	0	0.0	0	6	1
Mixed, frzn.	½ cup	59	12	1	3	0	0.0	0	32	4
Mushrooms										
can	½ cup	30	4	0	3	0	0.0	0	440	2
fried	5 medium	156	11	1	2	12	1.5	2	112	1
raw	½ cup	11	2	0	2	0	0.0	0	2	1
Okra, cooked	½ cup	18	4	0	2	0	0.0	0	5	2
Onions										
can	½ cup	21	5	0	1	0	0.0	0	416	1
chopped, raw	½ cup	32	8	½	1	0	0.0	0	3	1
rings, breaded & fried	5 medium	164	21	1 ½	2	9	2.0	0	321	1
Parsley, raw	¼ cup	5	1	0	0	0	0.0	0	8	1
Parsnips, cooked	½ cup	55	13	1	1	0	0.0	0	8	3
Pea pods, cooked	½ cup	34	6	½	3	0	0.0	0	3	2
Peas, green, cooked	½ cup	67	13	1	4	0	0.0	0	2	4

VEGETABLES

ITEM	AMOUNT	CALORIES	CARBOHYDRATE (g)	CARBOHYDRATE CHOICES	PROTEIN (g)	FAT (g)	SATURATED FAT (g)	CHOLESTEROL (mg)	SODIUM (mg)	FIBER (g)
Peppers, raw										
bell, green/red/yellow	½ cup	15	4	0	1	0	0.0	0	2	1
chiles, green, diced	2 T.	5	1	0	1	0	0.0	0	70	0
jalapeños	1 medium	4	1	0	0	0	0.0	0	0	0
Pierogies, potato, frzn.										
w/ cheese	3 (1.4 oz.)	180	34	2	6	3	1.0	5	530	1
w/o cheese	3 (1.4 oz.)	170	34	2	5	2	0.0	5	420	1
Pimentos, can	¼ cup	11	2	0	1	0	0.0	0	7	1
Potatoes, cooked										
au gratin, box	½ cup	114	17	1	2	4	1.0	2	510	1
baked, w/ skin	1 (4 oz.)	106	24	1 ½	3	0	0.0	0	11	3
blintzes, frzn.	1 (2.2 oz.)	90	15	1	3	4	1.0	5	170	2
boiled, w/o skin	1 (4 oz.)	98	23	1 ½	2	0	0.0	0	6	2
French fries, frzn.	14 medium	120	20	1	2	4	0.5	0	350	2
hash browns, frzn.	½ cup	106	15	1	2	4	0.5	0	0	1
instant, w/ margarine & milk	½ cup	140	19	1	3	6	1.0	2	234	2
knish, frzn.	1 (2 oz.)	200	19	1	4	12	2.5	55	130	1
mashed, w/ margarine & milk	½ cup	117	18	1	2	4	1.0	1	350	2
O'Brien, frzn.	½ cup	198	21	1 ½	2	13	3.0	0	42	2
pancakes, hmde.	1 medium	204	21	1 ½	5	11	2.0	72	581	2
scalloped, box	½ cup	130	22	1 ½	3	4	1.0	2	628	2
steak fries	7 medium	110	19	1	2	3	0.5	0	330	2
Tater Tots®, frzn.	9	170	20	1	2	8	1.5	0	420	2
twice baked, w/ cheese	1 (5 oz.)	193	27	2	4	8	2.5	0	466	3
Pumpkin, can	½ cup	42	10	½	1	0	0.0	0	6	4
Radishes, raw	10 medium	7	2	0	0	0	0.0	0	18	1
Rutabagas, cooked	½ cup	47	11	1	2	0	0.0	0	24	2
Salad greens, raw	1 cup	10	3	0	1	0	0.0	0	20	1
Sauerkraut, can	½ cup	22	5	0	1	0	0.0	0	780	3
Scallions, raw	1 T.	2	1	0	0	0	0.0	0	1	0
Shallots, raw	¼ cup	29	7	½	1	0	0.0	0	5	0
Spinach										
cooked	½ cup	21	3	0	3	0	0.0	0	63	2
creamed	½ cup	80	10	½	4	3	1.5	0	520	2
raw	1 cup	7	1	0	1	0	0.0	0	24	1
Squash										
acorn, cooked	½ cup	57	15	1	1	0	0.0	0	4	5
butternut, cooked	½ cup	47	12	1	2	0	0.0	0	2	3
spaghetti	½ cup	21	5	0	1	0	0.0	0	14	1
summer, cooked/raw	½ cup	18	4	0	1	0	0.0	0	1	1
winter, cooked	½ cup	38	9	½	1	0	0.0	0	1	3
zucchini, cooked	½ cup	14	4	0	1	0	0.0	0	3	1

VEGETABLES

ITEM	AMOUNT	CALORIES	CARBOHYDRATE (g)	CARBOHYDRATE CHOICES	PROTEIN (g)	FAT (g)	SATURATED FAT (g)	CHOLESTEROL (mg)	SODIUM (mg)	FIBER (g)
Squash *(continued)*										
zucchini, raw	½ cup	10	2	0	1	0	0.0	0	6	1
Succotash, cooked	½ cup	110	23	1 ½	5	1	0.0	0	16	4
Sweet potatoes										
baked, w skin	1 (4 oz.)	103	24	1 ½	2	0	0.0	0	41	4
candied, frzn.	½ cup	276	67	4 ½	1	1	0.5	0	109	3
mashed, w/o fat	½ cup	125	29	2	2	0	0.0	0	44	4
Swiss chard, cooked	½ cup	18	4	0	2	0	0.0	0	157	2
Tomatoes										
cherry, raw	6 medium	18	4	0	1	0	0.0	0	5	1
paste, can	½ cup	120	24	1 ½	8	0	0.0	0	80	4
puree, can	½ cup	48	11	1	2	0	0.0	0	499	2
stewed, can	½ cup	35	9	½	1	0	0.0	0	220	1
sun dried	½ cup	70	15	1	4	1	0.0	0	566	3
whole, can	½ cup	20	5	0	1	0	0.0	0	172	1
whole, raw	1 medium	27	6	½	1	0	0.0	0	7	2
Turnips, cooked	½ cup	25	6	½	1	0	0.0	0	18	2
Water chestnuts, can	½ cup	35	9	½	1	0	0.0	0	6	2
Watercress, raw	½ cup	2	0	0	0	0	0.0	0	7	0
Wax beans, cooked	½ cup	22	5	0	1	0	0.0	0	2	2
Yams, cooked										
baked, w/ skin	1 (4 oz.)	102	24	1 ½	2	0	0.0	0	41	4
mashed, w/o fat	½ cup	79	19	1	1	0	0.0	0	5	3

VEGETARIAN FOODS & LEGUMES

ITEM	AMOUNT	CALORIES	CARBOHYDRATE (g)	CARBOHYDRATE CHOICES	PROTEIN (g)	FAT (g)	SATURATED FAT (g)	CHOLESTEROL (mg)	SODIUM (mg)	FIBER (g)
Aduki/adzuki beans										
dry, cooked	½ cup	147	29	1 ½	9	0	0.0	0	9	8
sweetened, can	½ cup	351	81	5 ½	6	0	0.0	0	323	4
Bac-O's®										
bits	1 T.	30	2	0	3	2	0.0	0	120	0
chips	1½ T.	30	2	0	3	2	0.0	0	115	0
Bacon, vegetarian	2 (0.3 oz.)	60	2	0	2	5	0.5	0	230	1
Baked beans, vegetarian, can	½ cup	150	30	2	8	1	0.0	0	390	8
Black beans										
can	½ cup	110	17	1	7	1	0.0	0	400	7
dry, cooked	½ cup	114	20	1	8	1	0.0	0	1	8
Black eyed peas/cowpeas										
can	½ cup	92	16	1	6	1	0.0	0	359	4
dry, cooked	½ cup	80	17	1	3	0	0.0	0	3	4
Black turtle beans										
can	½ cup	109	20	1	7	0	0.0	0	461	8
dry, cooked	½ cup	120	23	1	8	0	0.0	0	3	5

VEGETARIAN FOODS & LEGUMES

ITEM	AMOUNT	CALORIES	CARBOHYDRATE (g)	CARBOHYDRATE CHOICES	PROTEIN (g)	FAT (g)	SATURATED FAT (g)	CHOLESTEROL (mg)	SODIUM (mg)	FIBER (g)
Boca®, burgers										
cheeseburger	1 (2.5 oz.)	100	6	½	13	5	1.5	10	320	4
grilled vegetable	1 (2.5 oz.)	80	7	½	12	1	0.0	0	300	4
original	1 (2.5 oz.)	70	6	½	13	1	0.0	0	280	4
vegan	1 (2.5 oz.)	100	9	½	13	3	0.0	0	470	4
Boca®, meatless products										
breakfast links										
chik'n nuggets	4 (0.8 oz.)	180	17	1	14	7	1.0	0	500	3
chik'n patties	1 (2.5 oz.)	160	15	1	11	6	0.0	0	430	2
ground crumbles	2 oz.	60	6	½	13	1	0.0	0	270	3
spicy chick'n patties	1 (2.5 oz.)	160	15	1	11	6	1.0	0	560	2
Broad/fava beans										
can	½ cup	110	20	1	6	1	0.0	0	250	5
dry, cooked	½ cup	94	17	1	7	0	0.0	0	4	5
Butter beans, can	½ cup	90	16	1	6	0	0.0	0	450	4
Calico beans, dry, cooked	½ cup	127	24	1	8	0	0.0	0	6	9
Cannellini beans, can	½ cup	100	18	1	5	1	0.0	0	270	5
Chickpeas/garbanzo beans										
can	½ cup	100	17	1	5	2	0.0	0	280	4
dry, cooked	½ cup	135	23	1	7	2	0.0	0	6	6
Chili, vegetarian, can	1 cup	205	38	2	12	1	0.0	0	778	10
Chili beans, can	½ cup	110	24	1	7	1	0.5	0	360	7
Cranberry/Roman beans										
can	½ cup	108	20	1	7	0	0.0	0	432	8
dry, cooked	½ cup	120	22	1	8	0	0.0	0	1	9
Crowder peas, can	½ cup	110	18	1	7	1	0.0	0	500	5
Falafel patties	1 (0.6 oz.)	57	5	0	2	3	0.5	0	50	1
Gardenburger®, burgers										
black bean chipotle	1 (2.5 oz.)	100	16	1	5	3	0.0	0	390	5
portabella	1 (2.5 oz.)	100	17	1	3	1	0.0	0	490	5
original	1 (2.5 oz.)	100	18	1	5	3	1.0	10	400	5
sun-dried tomato basil	1 (2.5 oz.)	100	17	1	4	3	0.5	0	270	4
Great Northern beans										
can	½ cup	70	17	1	6	0	0.0	0	490	6
dry, cooked	½ cup	104	19	1	7	0	0.0	0	2	6
Ground meat alternative	⅓ cup	60	5	0	10	1	0.0	0	270	2
Hot dogs										
tofu	1 (1.5 oz.)	60	2	0	8	3	0.5	0	300	1
veggie	1 (1.5 oz.)	45	3	0	8	0	0.0	0	290	0
Hummus	½ cup	218	25	1 ½	6	11	1.5	0	298	5
Kidney beans										
can	½ cup	108	19	1	7	0	0.0	0	379	6

VEGETARIAN FOODS & LEGUMES

ITEM	AMOUNT	CALORIES	CARBOHYDRATE (g)	CARBOHYDRATE CHOICES	PROTEIN (g)	FAT (g)	SATURATED FAT (g)	CHOLESTEROL (mg)	SODIUM (mg)	FIBER (g)
Kidney beans *(continued)*										
dry, cooked	½ cup	112	20	1	8	0	0.0	0	2	7
Lentils, cooked	½ cup	115	20	1	9	0	0.0	0	2	8
Lima beans										
baby, frzn.	½ cup	95	18	1	6	0	0.0	0	26	5
can	½ cup	95	18	1	6	0	0.0	0	405	6
dry, cooked	½ cup	108	20	1	7	0	0.0	0	2	7
Miso	2 T.	68	9	½	4	2	0.5	0	1282	2
Morningstar Farms®, burgers										
chipotle black bean	1 (4.2 oz.)	210	24	1 ½	17	7	1.0	0	700	2
garden veggie patties	1 (2.4 oz.)	110	9	½	10	4	0.5	0	350	3
Grillers® original	1 (2.3 oz.)	130	5	0	15	6	1.0	0	260	2
mushroom lover's	1 (2.3 oz.)	110	8	½	7	6	1.0	0	220	1
Morningstar Farms®, meatless products										
bacon, egg & cheese biscuit	1 (3.7 oz.)	270	40	2 ½	9	8	4.0	25	630	1
Buffalo wings	5 (0.3 oz.)	200	20	1	12	8	1.0	0	640	3
chik'n nuggets	4 (0.8 oz.)	190	19	1	12	9	1.5	0	600	4
chik'n tenders	2 (1.4 oz.)	190	20	1	12	7	1.0	0	580	3
Mung beans, dry, cooked	½ cup	106	19	1	7	0	0.0	0	2	8
Natto	½ cup	186	13	½	16	10	1.5	0	6	5
Navy beans										
can	½ cup	148	27	1 ½	10	1	0.0	0	587	7
dry, cooked	½ cup	127	24	1	8	1	0.0	0	0	10
Pigeon peas										
can	½ cup	70	14	1	4	0	0.0	0	390	4
dry, cooked	½ cup	102	20	1	6	0	0.0	0	4	6
Pink beans, dry, cooked	½ cup	126	24	1 ½	8	0	0.0	0	2	5
Pinto beans										
can	½ cup	103	18	1	6	1	0.0	0	353	6
dry, cooked	½ cup	122	22	1	8	1	0.0	0	1	8
Red beans, dry, cooked	½ cup	122	23	1	8	0	0.0	0	6	9
Refried beans, can										
fat free	½ cup	100	18	1	6	0	0.0	0	580	6
regular	½ cup	150	25	1	8	3	1.0	0	570	9
Sausages, vegetarian										
ground	2 oz.	60	8	½	7	0	0.0	0	490	2
links	1 (1 oz.)	50	4	0	5	2	0.5	0	290	2
patties	1 (1 oz.)	40	2	0	6	1	0.0	0	175	1
Seitan		227	21	1 ½	32	2	0.0	0	30	3
chicken-style	5 oz.	110	4	0	20	2	0.0	0	770	2
stir-fry strips	3 oz.	110	2	0	22	2	0.0	0	420	1
traditional	3 oz.	90	3	0	18	1	0.0	0	380	1

VEGETARIAN FOODS & LEGUMES

ITEM	AMOUNT	CALORIES	CARBOHYDRATE (g)	CARBOHYDRATE CHOICES	PROTEIN (g)	FAT (g)	SATURATED FAT (g)	CHOLESTEROL (mg)	SODIUM (mg)	FIBER (g)
Soy meal, defatted	½ cup	206	22	1	30	1	0.0	0	2	11
Soy protein										
concentrate	1 oz.	94	9	½	17	0	0.0	0	1	2
isolate	1 oz.	96	2	0	23	1	0.0	0	285	2
Soybeans										
green, cooked	½ cup	127	10	½	11	6	0.5	0	13	4
mature, cooked	½ cup	149	9	½	14	8	1.0	0	1	5
mature, roasted, salted	¼ cup	203	14	½	15	11	1.5	0	70	8
Split peas, dry, cooked	½ cup	116	21	1	8	0	0.0	0	2	8
Tempeh										
flax	4 oz.	220	16	½	20	9	1.5	0	0	11
soy	4 oz.	230	16	½	22	8	1.0	0	10	12
wild rice	4 oz.	230	22	1	19	8	1.0	0	5	12
Tofu										
firm, lite	2.8 oz.	40	1	0	7	2	0.0	0	25	0
firm, regular	2.8 oz.	70	2	0	7	3	0.0	0	0	0
flavored, baked	3 oz.	90	3	0	8	5	1.0	0	250	1
silken, lite	3.2 oz.	30	0	0	6	1	0.0	0	65	0
silken, regular	3.2 oz.	45	1	0	4	2	0.0	0	0	0
soft, regular	3 oz.	60	1	0	6	3	0.0	0	0	0
Tofurky®, meatless products										
breakfast links	1 (1.6 oz.)	120	6	½	10	6	0.0	0	320	2
deli slices	5 (0.4 oz.)	100	6	½	13	3	0.0	0	300	3
franks	1 (1.6 oz.)	80	5	0	11	2	0.0	0	390	3
jurky	4 (0.5 oz.)	100	9	½	12	2	0.0	0	260	1
Turkey style slices	4 (0.5 oz.)	100	5	0	13	4	0.5	0	300	2
TVP®, dry	¼ cup	80	7	½	12	0	0.0	0	2	4
White beans, dry, cooked	½ cup	124	23	1	9	0	0.0	0	5	6
Winged beans, dry, cooked	½ cup	126	13	1	9	5	0.5	0	11	2
Yeast										
Brewer's, buds/flakes	3 T.	116	13	½	16	0	0.0	0	63	6
nutritional, flakes	3 T.	60	12	1	7	0	0.0	0	2	4
nutritional, powder	3 T.	54	6	½	7	4	0.0	0	18	4

Favorite Foods

ITEM	AMOUNT	CALORIES	CARBOHYDRATE (g)	CARBOHYDRATE CHOICES	PROTEIN (g)	FAT (g)	SATURATED FAT (g)	CHOLESTEROL (mg)	SODIUM (mg)	FIBER (g)

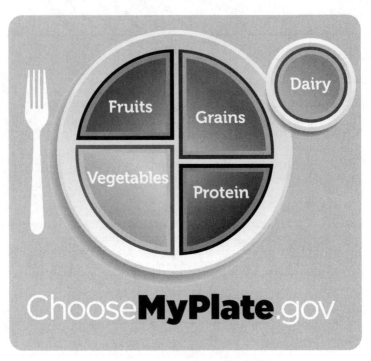

MyPlate is part of an overall food guidance system that emphasizes a personalized plan to eat healthfully. MyPlate helps individuals use the Dietary Guidelines to make smart choices from every food group, find balance between food and physical activity, get the most nutrition out of calories, and stay within daily calorie needs.

Additional information about USDA's MyPlate is available at **ChooseMyPlate.gov**. The latest Dietary Guidelines for Americans and a description of a healthy diet for the general public over 2 years of age is available at **www.choosemyplate.gov/guidelines/index.html**.

Estimate your Daily Nutrient Goals in Three Easy Steps

Step 1

Determine your recommended calorie goal using the information below. If you want to lose between one-half to one pound per week, subtract 250-500 calories from the recommended ranges. For a balanced diet, women should not eat less than 1200 calories and men should not eat less than 1500 calories each day.

1500-1800 calories
Sedentary women and some older adults

1800-2400 calories
Active women and many sedentary men

2400-2800 calories
Active men and some very active women

Step 2

Locate your calorie goal on the left-hand side of the chart below. Read the chart across to the right to determine your other nutrient goals. Each nutrient goal is based on a percentage of your calorie goal. Three different levels for fat and two levels for saturated fat goals are listed. Your goal is to eat within the recommended ranges.

Step 3

Look at the bottom of the chart for cholesterol, sodium and fiber recommendations. If you have special nutrient needs, talk with your health care provider or registered dietitian for the amounts that are right for you.

Calorie Goal	Fat Grams			Saturated Fat Grams		Carbohydrate Grams	Protein Grams
	30%	25%	20%	10%	7%	50-60%	10-15%
1200	40	33	27	13	9	150-180	30-45
1500	50	42	33	17	12	188-225	38-56
1800	60	50	40	20	14	225-270	45-68
2000	67	56	44	22	16	250-300	50-75
2200	73	61	49	24	17	275-330	55-83
2500	83	69	56	28	19	313-375	63-94
2800	93	78	62	31	22	350-420	70-105

Cholesterol	Sodium	Fiber
300 milligrams	2400 milligrams	25 to 35 grams

If you have diabetes and are counting carbohydrate grams or carbohydrate choices, each has been provided for you in this book. The amount of carbohydrate grams and choices you can eat is based on your calorie goal.

Carbohydrate Goals for Diabetes

Calorie Goal	Carbohydrate Grams	Carbohydrate Choices
1200	150-180	10-12
1500	188-225	13-15
1800	225-270	15-18
2000	250-300	17-20
2200	275-330	18-22
2500	313-375	21-25
2800	350-420	23-28

Carbohydrate choices have been calculated using the 15-Gram Equation (15 grams of carbohydrate = 1 carbohydrate choice). We have done the calculating for you for all foods listed in this book. Since fiber is part of the total carbohydrate, when fiber was 5 grams or greater, half of it was subtracted from the total carbohydrate grams before calculating carbohydrate choices.

Carbohydrate Grams	Carbohydrate Choices
0-5	0
6-10	½
11-20	1
21-25	1½
26-35	2
36-40	2½
41-50	3
51-55	3½
56-65	4
66-70	4½
71-80	5

Looking for an Individualized Eating Plan?

A registered dietitian (RD) can help. To locate an RD in your area, contact the Academy of Nutrition and Dietetics (formerly known as The American Dietetics Association) referral service by calling 1-800-366-1655 or visit the website at **www.eatright.org**.

Desirable Levels:
Blood Lipids & Blood Pressure

	General Population	Diabetes	Coronary Heart Disease
Cholesterol	<200 mg/dL	<200 mg/dL	<180 mg/dL
LDL	<100 mg/dL	<100 mg/dL	<70-100 mg/dL
HDL	>40 mg/dL (men) >50 mg/dL (women)	>45 mg/dL (men) >55 mg/dL (women)	>55 mg/dL
Triglycerides	<150 mg/dL	<150 mg/dL	<150 mg/dL
Blood Pressure	<120/80 mmHg	<130/80 mmHg	<120/80 mmHg

Source: National Heart, Lung & Blood Institute. Adult Treatment III Guidelines.
http://www.nhlbi.nih.gov/guidelines/cholesterol/atp3upd04.htm.
Accessed October 14, 2011.

Goals

Cholesterol: _____

LDL: _____

HDL: _____

Triglycerides: _____

Blood Pressure: _____

Weight: _____

Know Your Numbers

Date	Cholesterol	LDL	HDL	Triglycerides	Blood Pressure	Weight	Other/Comments

Medications/Supplements

Start Date	Name of Medication & Dosage	Comments	Stop Date

References

Books and Periodicals

AADE. "Carbohydrate-Counting Skills" and "Challenges and Advantages of Carbohydrate Counting." In *The Art and Science of Diabetes Self-Management Education Desk Reference*, Second edition. Chicago: American Association of Diabetes Educators; 2010.

American College of Sports Medicine. *ACSM's Resource Manual for Guidelines for Exercise Testing and Prescription*, Sixth edition. Philadelphia: Lippincott, Williams & Wilkins; 2009.

American Diabetes Association. *Clinical Practice Recommendations 2010*. The American Diabetes Association; 2010.

American Diabetes Association and The American Dietetic Association. *Choose Your Foods: Exchange Lists for Diabetes*; ADA Publication; 2008.

Parker, Suzi. *1000 Best Bartender's Recipes*. Illinois: Sourcebooks, Inc.; 2005.

Other

- Fast food franchise nutrition information, 2011.

- Manufacturer's Nutrition Facts food labels, 2011.

- The Food Processor, Nutrition & Fitness Software. Salem, OR: ESHA Research, 2011.

- National Cholesterol Education Program Report. Implications of Recent Clinical Trials for the National Cholesterol Education Program (NCEP) Adult Treatment III Guidelines. **http://www.nhlbi.nih.gov/guidelines/cholesterol/atp3upd04.htm**. Accessed October 14, 2011.

- USDA's MyPlate. **http://www.choosemyplate.gov**. Accessed November 1, 2011.

- USDA's MyPlate.gov – Dietary Guidelines for Americans. **http://www.choosemyplate.gov/guidelines/index.html**. Accessed November 1, 2011.

- U.S. Dept of Health and Human Services. The Seventh Report of the Joint National Committee on Prevention, Detection, Evaluation, and Treatment of High Blood Pressure (JNC7). **http://www.nhlbi.nih.gov/guidelines/hypertension**. Accessed October 18, 2011.

Calories Used Through Activity

Listed below are the number of calories used during 30 minutes of various activities. Calorie values are approximate and vary based on an individual's weight, exertion and skill level. Values were calculated for a 150-pound person. To adjust for your weight: divide your weight by 150, then multiply this number (your weight factor) by the calorie values on this chart.

Activity	30 minutes
Aerobic dance	215
Archery	125
Badminton	161
Baseball/softball	179
Basketball	215
Bicycling, <10 mph	143
Bicycling, 10-12 mph	215
Bicycling, >12 mph	287
Bowling	107
Boxing/sparring	322
Canoeing	125
Dancing	161
Farming, driving tractor	89
Fencing	215
Fishing	143
Football	287
Gardening	179
Golfing, w cart	125
Golfing, w/o cart	161
Golfing, walk & carry clubs	197

Activity	30 minutes
Handball	430
Hiking	215
Hockey, field/ice	287
Horseback riding	143
Housework/cleaning	125
Hunting	179
Ice skating	251
Judo/karate	358
Jumping rope	358
Kayaking	179
Kick boxing/tae kwon do	358
Mountain biking	304
Mountain/rock climbing	287
Mowing lawn	197
Painting, outside	179
Pool (billiards)	89
Racquetball	251
Roller blading/skating	251
Rowing machine	341
Running, 5mph	287

Calories Used Through Activity *(continued)*

Activity	30 minutes
Running, 8mph	483
Running, 10mph	573
Sailing	107
Scuba diving	251
Sitting	36
Ski machine	340
Skiing, cross-country, 4-5 mph.	287
Skiing, downhill	215
Sleeping	32
Snow shoeing	287
Snow shoveling	215
Soccer	251
Squash	430
Stair climbing	330
Standing	43
Stationary bike	179

Activity	30 minutes
Stretching	143
Swimming, fast	358
Swimming, slow	287
Table tennis (ping pong)	143
Tai chi	143
Tennis, doubles	215
Tennis, singles	287
Treading water	143
Volleyball	107
Walking, 3 mph.	125
Walking, 4 mph.	143
Water aerobics	143
Water-skiing	215
Weight training (moderate)	107
Weight training (vigorous)	215
Wrestling	215
Yoga	143

Index

HealthCheques™: A Self-Monitoring System

by Jane Stephenson, RD, CDE, and Diane Bader. Copyright 2012. Track calories, fat, carbohydrates, carb choices, protein, saturated fat, sodium, cholesterol or fiber on a daily basis using this easy-to-carry checkbook. Each checkbook set consists of a 112-page Food Counter that provides nutrient values for more than 1,500 foods. The lower portion is a Food & Activity Log to record the foods eaten and physical activity. Replace the Log as needed.

Diet-Free HealthCheques™: A Self-Enrichment System

by Jane Stephenson, RD, CDE and Jackie Boucher, MS, RD, CDE. Copyright 2000. An ideal system for those who do not need another "diet", yet want to enjoy food without guilt. Designed for the chronic dieter, binge eater, and stress eater, this tool focuses on 10 S.T.R.A.T.E.G.I.E.S. that give the individual the "why" and "how" behind developing a healthier relationship with food, self, activity, and weight. The 4-week Journal on the lower portion helps the individual track eating and activity habits, identify common feelings and situations that 'trigger' problematic eating behavior, and gauge satiety levels. Replace the Journal as needed.

HealthCheques™: A Meal-Planning System

by Jane Stephenson, RD, CDE. Copyright 2010. This meal-planning tool lets you decide what, how much, and when to eat. A full set includes the Food Exchange Guide, which lists all foods categorized by the six major Exchange Lists and a 4-week Food and Activity Journal. The Guide has extensive Fast Foods, Restaurant Foods, and Mixed Dishes sections. The Journal allows you to record blood glucose levels and all foods and beverages eaten throughout the day. Also provided is an easy checkbox system of tracking food exchanges, with room to record grams of carbohydrate and physical activity expended. Included are sample meal plans ranging from 1200 to 3000 calories, plus room to add your own individualized food plan. Replace the Journal as needed.

Any of the above sets can be ordered on page 137. Please call our toll-free number (800-322-5679) if you have any questions or visit **www.appletree-press.com**.

REORDER FORM and Other Products from Appletree Press!

HealthCheques™ checkbook sets:
(see page 136 for product description)

A) **HealthCheques™: A Self-Monitoring System**
by Jane Stephenson, RD, CDE and Diane Bader
Copyright 2012.
Item #400   **$9.25 each: Send me _____ at $_____ .**

B) **Diet-Free HealthCheques™: A Self-Enrichment System**
by Jane Stephenson, RD, CDE and Jackie Boucher, MS, RD, CDE.
Copyright 2000.
Item #420   **$7.95 each: Send me _____ at $_____ .**

C) **HealthCheques™: A Meal-Planning System**
by Jane Stephenson, RD, CDE.
Copyright 2010.
Item #430   **$8.95 each: Send me _____ at $_____ .**

HealthCheques™: Carbohydrate, Fat & Calorie Guide
Fourth Edition
by Jane Stephenson, RD, CDE and Diane Bader.

Softcover, 140 pages. Copyright 2013. A comprehensive pocket guide listing the calories, carbohydrate, protein, fat, saturated fat, cholesterol, sodium and fiber content of 4,500 foods. Includes carbohydrate choices.

**$7.95 each:
Send me _____ at $_____ .**

SHIPPING INFORMATION:

Add: $4.00 for one book or checkbook

$5.00 for two books or book & checkbook $ _____

(Minnesota residents must add sales tax) 7.38% tax $ _____

TOTAL ENCLOSED $ _____

Circle Method of Payment: Check   Visa   MasterCard

Card Number _____ Expiration Date _____

Name _____

P.O. Box and/or Street Address_____

_____

City, State and Zip Code _____

MAIL TO: **Appletree Press, Inc.**   Toll-free: 1-800-322-5679
Suite 125   Fax: (507) 345-3002
151 Good Counsel Drive   Phone: (507) 345-4848
Mankato, MN 56001   Website: www.appletree-press.com